W9-BLR-776

Coronary Artery Disease

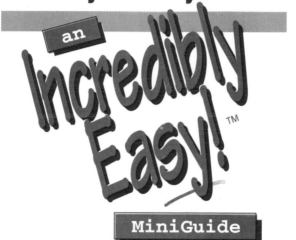
an Incredibly Easy!™

MiniGuide

Coronary Artery Disease

an Incredibly Easy!™

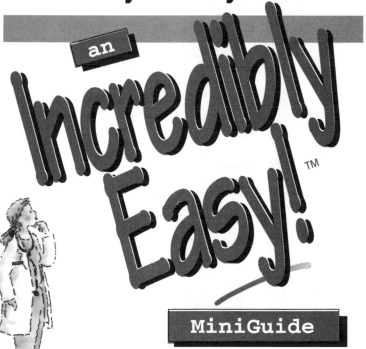

MiniGuide

Springhouse Corporation
Springhouse, Pennsylvania

Staff

Vice President
Matthew Cahill

Clinical Director
Judith A. Schilling McCann, RN, MSN

Art Director
John Hubbard

Executive Editor
Michael Shaw

Managing Editor
Andrew T. McPhee, RN, BSN

Clinical Editors
Collette Hendler, RN, CCRN; Jill M. Curry, RN, BSN, CCRN; Joan M. Robinson, RN, MSN, CCRN; Carla M. Roy, RN, BSN, CCRN

Editors
Kevin Haworth, Anna Wahrman

Copy Editors
Brenna H. Mayer (manager), Gretchen Fee, Stacey A. Follin, Pamela Wingrod

Designers
Arlene Putterman (associate art director), Mary Ludwicki (book designer), Joseph John Clark, Donna Morris

Illustrators
Bot Roda, Jacalyn B. Facciolo

Typography
Diane Paluba (manager), Joyce Rossi Biletz, Valerie Molettiere

Manufacturing
Deborah Meiris (director), Patricia K. Dorshaw, Otto Mezei (book production manager)

Editorial Assistants
Beverly Lane, Marcia Mills, Liz Schaeffer

Indexer
Ellen Murray

Printed in the United States of America.

IEMCAD-010899

Ⓡ A member of the Reed Elsevier plc group

Library of Congress Cataloging-in-Publication Data

Coronary Artery Disease: an incredibly easy miniguide
  p. cm. – (Incredibly easy miniguide)
  Includes index.
  1. Coronary heart disease handbooks, manuals, etc. 2. Coronary heart disease—Nursing handbooks, manuals, etc.
  I. Springhouse Corporation.
  II. Series.
[DNLM: 1.Coronary Disease Handbooks. WG 39 C821 1999]
RC865.C6C6313 1999
616.1'23—dc21
DNLM/DLC   99-25003
ISBN 1-58255-013-1 (alk. paper)   CIP

Contents

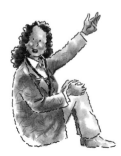

v

Contributors and consultants

Joanne M. Bartelmo, RN, MSN, CCRN
Clinical Educator
Pottstown (Pa.) Memorial Medical Center

Nancy Cirone, RN,C, MSN, CDE
Director of Education
Warminster (Pa.) Hospital

Margaret Friant Cramer, RN, MSN
Clinical Supervisor
Cardiac Solutions, Inc.
Fort Washington, Pa.

Michael Carter, RN, DNSc, FAAN
Dean and Professor
College of Nursing
University of Tennessee
Memphis

Pamela Mullen Kovach, RN, BSN
Independent Clinical Consultant
Perkiomenville, Pa.

Patricia A. Lange, RN, MSN, CS, CCRN, EdD (candidate)
Graduate Nursing Program Coordinator and Assistant Professor of Nursing
Hawaii Pacific University
Kaneohe

Mary Ann Siciliano McLaughlin, RN, MSN
Clinical Supervisor
Cardiac Solutions, Inc.
Fort Washington, Pa.

Lori Musolf Neri, RN, MSN, CCRN
Clinical Instructor
Villanova (Pa.) University

Joseph L. Neri, DO, FACC
Cardiologist
The Heart Care Group
Allentown, Pa.

Robert Rauch
Manager of Government Relations
Amgen, Inc.
Thousand Oaks, Calif.

Larry E. Simmons, RN, PhD (candidate)
Clinical Instructor
University of Missouri-Kansas City

Foreword

More than 5 million people in the United States are known to have coronary artery disease (CAD). CAD causes more deaths among adult men and women than any other disorder. It occurs most often in middle-aged or elderly white men. More than 50% of men age 60 and older show signs of CAD, making CAD the most common form of heart disease in the nation.

Meeting the challenges of caring for a patient with CAD requires a full understanding of the disorder and its implications for care. At once accurate, authoritative, and completely up-to-date, *Coronary Artery Disease: An Incredibly Easy MiniGuide* can help you gain an in-depth understanding of CAD in an amazingly fun and exciting way.

The first chapter, *Understanding CAD,* lays the foundation for your understanding by providing basic facts about the pathophysiology of CAD and the effects of CAD on the body. The next three chapters cover prevention, assessment, and treatment of CAD. The fifth chapter covers complications of the disorder, and the final chapter covers patient teaching.

Throughout the book, you'll find features designed to make learning about CAD lively and entertaining. For instance, *Memory joggers* provide clever tricks for remembering key points. *Checklists,* rendered in the style of a classroom chalkboard, provide at-a-glance summaries of important facts.

Cartoon characters that nearly pop off the page provide light-hearted chuckles as well as reinforcement of essential material. And a *Quick quiz* at the end of every chapter gives you a chance to assess your learning and refresh your memory at the same time. The depth of information contained in this truly pocket-sized guide will impress even the most experienced health care professional. If you want a quick-learn, comprehensive reference about one of the most common conditions encountered in health care, I can't think of a more fitting resource than *Coronary Artery Disease: An Incredibly Easy MiniGuide.* It packs a wallop.

Michael Carter, RN, DNSc, FAAN
Dean and Professor
College of Nursing
University of Tennessee
Memphis

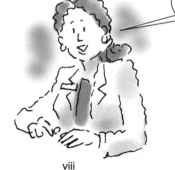

Professional development that's fun and exciting? Incredible!

Understanding CAD

Key facts

♦ Coronary artery disease (CAD) is a leading cause of death among men and women, particularly after age 60.

♦ CAD most commonly stems from atherosclerosis, a buildup of fatty tissue in the arteries.

♦ CAD develops progressively and may have a long latency period.

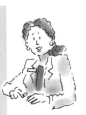

What is coronary artery disease?

Coronary artery disease (CAD), also known as coronary heart disease or atherosclerotic heart disease, is the most common form of heart disease in the United States. CAD causes more deaths among adult men and women than any other disorder. It occurs most commonly in middle-aged or elderly white men. More than 50% of men age 60 and older have obvious signs and symptoms of CAD.

Caution! Blocked artery ahead

In CAD, the coronary arteries become narrow or blocked, decreasing blood flow to the heart. This diminished flow deprives the heart of vital oxygen and nutrients, causing tissue damage and potentially serious complications.

CAD causes

Atherosclerosis is the most common cause of CAD. (See *Common causes of CAD.*) In this condition, fatty, fibrous plaques, possibly including calcium deposits, progressively narrow the coronary artery lumens, which reduces the volume of blood that can flow through them. This can lead to myocardial ischemia.

Risk factors you can't control

The risk of myocardial infarction (MI) as a result of CAD increases with the number of risk factors present. Some factors are controllable

Egad, this CAD really chokes me up. I receive less blood because arteries narrow or block up completely.

Now I get it!

Common causes of CAD
Numerous conditions can predispose a person to the development of CAD, including those listed here.

Cause	Description
Chlamydial infection	Some studies suggest that *Chlamydia* may be responsible for the development of CAD. No definitive studies are available.
Congenital coronary vascular defects	Examples include atrial and ventricular septal defects, coarctation of the aorta, and tetralogy of Fallot.
Coronary artery spasm	This spontaneous, sustained contraction of one or more coronary arteries causes ischemia and dysfunction of the heart muscle. It occurs in conjunction with atherosclerosis, though it can occur without it.
Dissecting aneurysm	The inner lining of the aorta or coronary artery tears and creates a new channel for blood to flow. It can eventually lead to the artery closing off completely.
Syphilis	About 10 to 25 years after an untreated infection, an aneurysm of the aorta or the leaking of an aortic valve may develop, impeding blood flow to the heart.
Vasculitis	The blood vessels that supply the heart become inflamed. The vessels then become weak or clogged, impairing blood flow to the heart.

and some aren't. (See *Risk factors and CAD,* page 6.) Uncontrollable risk factors include:

- being over age 40
- being male
- being white
- having a family history of CAD.

Risk factors you *can* control

Controllable CAD risk factors include:

- diabetes mellitus, especially in women
- inactivity
- increased low-density and decreased high-density lipoprotein levels

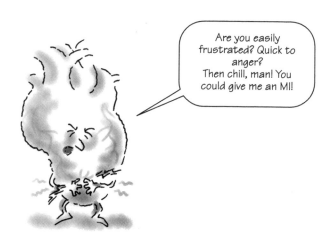

Are you easily frustrated? Quick to anger? Then chill, man! You could give me an MI!

• obesity, which increases the risk of diabetes mellitus, hypertension, and high cholesterol
• smoking (risk dramatically drops within 1 year of quitting)
• tendency to react to situations with anger or frustration
• systolic blood pressure greater than 160 mm Hg or diastolic blood pressure greater than 95 mm Hg.

Other risk factors

Other risk factors that can be modified include:
• elevated hematocrit
• environment (higher incidence of CAD in urban populations than rural populations)
• high resting heart rate
• increased levels of serum fibrinogen and uric acid
• natural or surgical menopause without estrogen replacement
• reduced vital capacity
• thyrotoxicosis
• use of oral contraceptives.

Risk factors and CAD

The more risk factors present, the greater the risk of myocardial infarction as a result of CAD. This chart, based on the famous Framingham Heart Study, shows how the risk increases with the number of risk factors present. The chart uses a systolic blood pressure of 180 mm Hg and a cholesterol level of 310 mg/dl in a 45-year-old man as a basis. The average risk level is 100.

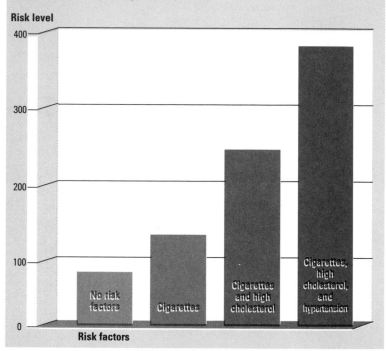

Risk level

Less common causes

Other factors that can reduce blood flow include congenital defects in the coronary vascular system, dissecting aneurysm, infectious vasculitis, and syphilis.

Coronary artery spasms

Coronary artery spasms can also impede blood flow. These spontaneous, sustained contractions of one or more coronary arteries occlude the vessel, reduce blood flow to the myocardium, and cause angina pectoris. Without treatment, ischemia and, eventually, MI result.

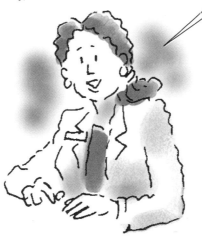

A spasm in a coronary artery can also interfere with blood flow and cause myocardial damage.

Slow flow problem

In its later stages, atherosclerosis can slow the flow of blood through coronary arteries in any of the following ways:

• Plaques (fatty deposits) obstruct the artery.
• Blood clots form around the plaques.
• Hemorrhages form in the damaged vessel walls beneath the plaques.
• Hardened vessels fail to dilate properly.

When a plaque ruptures

A plaque rupture, also known as an intimal tear or a plaque fissure, is a disruption in the plaque's surface. These disruptions create a channel uniting plaque lipids and blood products in the vessel lumen.

Contact between plaque lipids and blood products can cause a clot to form over the crack. If the clot becomes large enough, the patient could experience:

• unstable angina
• acute MI
• sudden death.

(Text continues on page 17.)

Cardiac anatomy

To understand the pathophysiology of CAD, you must first understand normal heart anatomy. The heart contains four chambers and four valves. The illustration below shows the major anatomic components of the heart.

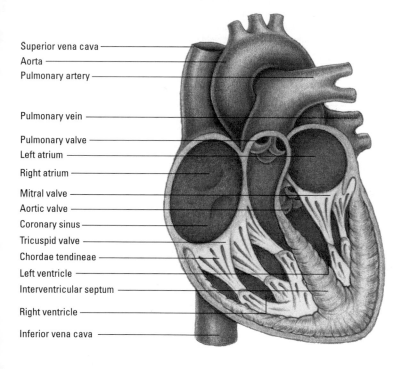

Superior vena cava
Aorta
Pulmonary artery

Pulmonary vein

Pulmonary valve
Left atrium
Right atrium

Mitral valve
Aortic valve
Coronary sinus
Tricuspid valve
Chordae tendineae
Left ventricle
Interventricular septum

Right ventricle

Inferior vena cava

Cardiac blood supply

The myocardium receives blood through four main coronary arteries, shown below. The circumflex artery supplies the left ventricle's lateral and posterior portions. The left anterior descending artery supplies the anterior wall of the left ventricle, the anterior interventricular septum, and the bundle branches. The right coronary artery supplies the sinoatrial and atrioventricular nodes, the right atrium and ventricle, and the inferior wall of the left ventricle. The posterior descending coronary artery supplies the left ventricle's posterior and inferior wall and the right ventricle's posterior wall.

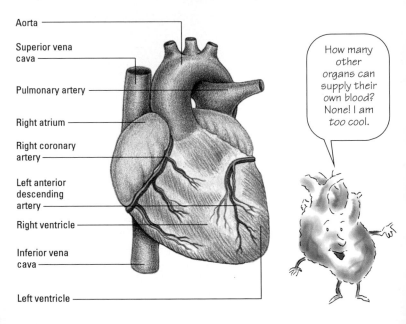

Inside the coronary arteries

There are three layers of a coronary artery — the tunica adventitia (outermost support-ing layer), tunica media (made up of a thin, fibrous lining), and the tunica intima (lined with endothelium, a thin layer of fibrous cells). The tunica intima regulates the activity and integrity of the coronary vasculature by secreting chemical mediators. Injury to this layer can initiate atherosclerotic plaque formation.

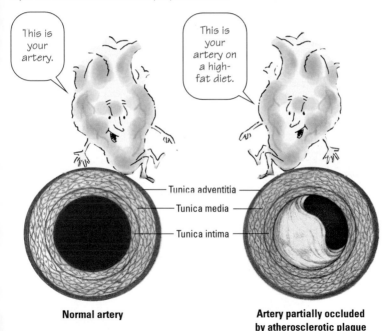

Normal artery

Artery partially occluded by atherosclerotic plaque

Development of atherosclerosis

CAD most commonly results from atherosclerosis. In atherosclerosis, fatty, fibrous plaques develop inside the arteries.
These plaques progressively narrow the arterial lumen, reducing the volume of blood that can flow through it and potentially
leading to myocardial ischemia (injury) or infarction (death).

Atherosclerosis evolves slowly, in many cases beginning in
childhood and progressing at different rates through adulthood. The evolution of atherosclerosis follows a typical path
and involves four stages.

Stage 1

The first stage, injury (shown below), starts with damage to
the tunica intima, which makes the arterial wall permeable to
circulating lipoproteins.

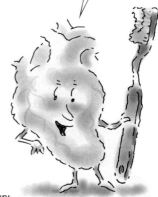

My arteries
must be kept
clean.
Otherwise a
great big
plaque may
develop.

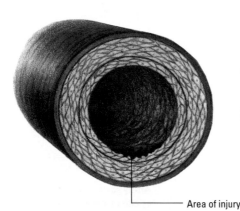

Area of injury

Development of atherosclerosis *(continued)*

Stage 2

In the next stage, lipoproteins invade smooth-muscle cells in the tunica intima, forming a nonobstructive lesion called a fatty streak.

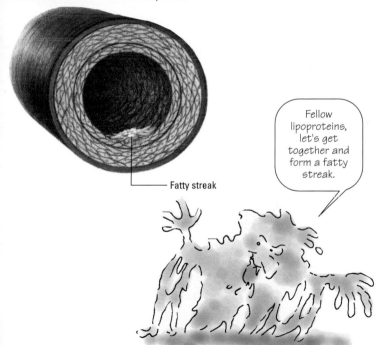

Fatty streak

Fellow lipoproteins, let's get together and form a fatty streak.

Development of atherosclerosis *(continued)*

Stage 3

In the acute, disruptive stage, a complicated lesion marked by calcification or rupture of the fibrous plaque appears. Thrombosis can occur, resulting in nearly total occlusion of the arterial lumen.

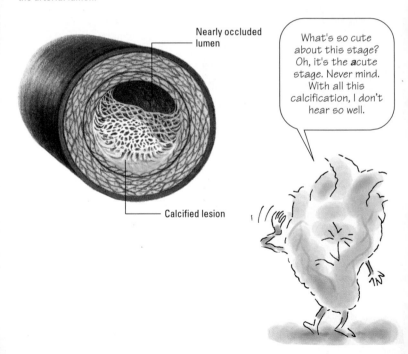

Nearly occluded lumen

Calcified lesion

Development of atherosclerosis *(continued)*

Stage 4

In the advanced stage, a fibrous plaque eventually develops and obstructs blood flow. Fibrous plaques contain lipoprotein-filled smooth-muscle cells, collagen, and muscle fibers.

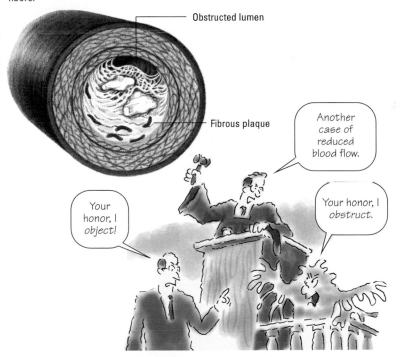

Restenosis and eccentric plaques

After angioplasty of an artery with an eccentric plaque, spasm can occur in the arclike, disease-free area. An eccentric plaque involves one side of the arterial lumen, leaving a slitlike or semilunar shaped lumen. During angioplasty, the disease-free wall may stretch without affecting the plaque. When the vessel wall relaxes, the lumen narrows, possibly leading to restenosis.

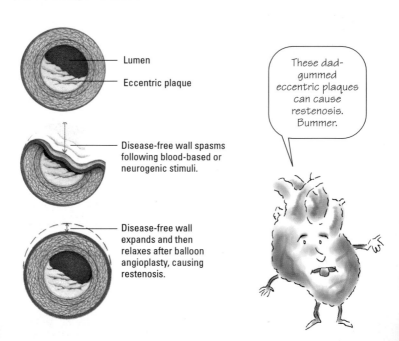

Lumen

Eccentric plaque

Disease-free wall spasms following blood-based or neurogenic stimuli.

Disease-free wall expands and then relaxes after balloon angioplasty, causing restenosis.

These dad-gummed eccentric plaques can cause restenosis. Bummer.

Turbulence and plaques

Plaques usually arise in areas of turbulent blood flow, where decreased artery diameter and elevated blood pressure favor plaque formation.

Quick quiz

1. Atherosclerosis can begin to develop during:

    A. childhood.
    B. adolescence.
    C. early adulthood.

Answer: A. The aorta can develop fatty streaks as early as childhood, though the patient typically remains asymptomatic until late middle-age.

2. The first step in plaque formation occurs when:

    A. smooth muscle cells proliferate in the area.
    B. the artery's endothelial layer suffers damage.
    C. a blood clot forms on the epithelial layer.

Answer: B. Most studies suggest that plaque formation begins after the endothelial layer suffers damage.

3. Potential causes of CAD include:
  A. chronic hepatitis.
  B. syphilis.
  C. viral myocarditis.

Answer: B. Of the diseases mentioned, only syphilis is known to lead to CAD.

4. Plaque rupture can lead to:
  A. heart failure.
  B. cerebrovascular accident.
  C. MI.

Answer: C. Rupture of an atherosclerotic plaque can lead to acute MI, unstable angina, or even sudden death.

Scoring

☆☆☆ If you answered all four questions correctly, super! You don't have any blockages, and your learning is flowing freely!

☆☆ If you answered three questions correctly, good job! You're nearly ready to earn a plaque for learning about plaque!

☆ If you answered fewer than three questions correctly, not to worry. A little angioplasty on your learning curve, and you'll be as good as new!

2

Preventing CAD

> ### Key facts
> ♦ CAD affects both sexes but emerges later in women than in men.
> ♦ Many risk factors, modifiable and nonmodifiable, may make patients vulnerable to atherosclerosis and CAD.
> ♦ Even after CAD develops, reducing risk factors can help control long-term problems related to CAD.

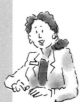

Who's at risk for CAD?

CAD occurs more commonly among men than women, and more commonly among whites than blacks. After menopause, however, women develop CAD at the same rate as men.

Don't wait for symptoms

Patients can live with CAD for years before they show signs and symptoms of the disease. Early treatment of CAD involves identifying patients at risk and taking steps to slow the development of CAD before symptoms arise.

By identifying patients with significant risk factors, treatment can begin before the patient suffers serious CAD-related complications.

Identifying risk factors

Factors that put people at risk for developing CAD can be categorized in two groups:

☝ nonmodifiable risk factors (those that can't be changed or controlled)

✌ modifiable risk factors (those that can be changed or controlled).

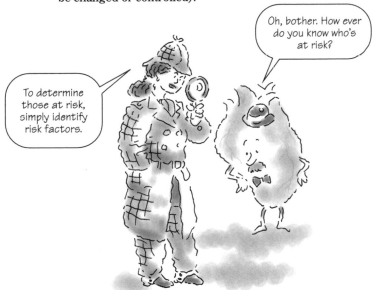

Nonmodifiable risk factors

Because nonmodifiable risk factors can't be changed, early identification of patients with these risk factors can help make treatment of the disease more effective. Nonmodifiable risk factors include:
- family history
- gender
- race
- age.

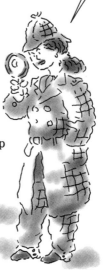

Look first for a family history of CAD.

All in the family

A person with a family history of CAD or hyperlipidemia faces an increased risk of developing CAD. Determine your patient's family history of CAD, going as far back in time as possible, to help determine his level of risk.

CAD hits men hard...

CAD strikes men particularly hard. Men suffer from CAD more commonly than women do, and men over age 40 are more likely to die of complications of CAD than of any other disease. CAD also permanently disables more men under age 65 than any other condition.

...but women don't escape CAD

After about age 50, women become just as likely as men to develop CAD. In addition, CAD takes a more complicated course in women, making the condition harder to treat after it has been identified. (See *Women and CAD,* page 24.)

A matter of race

CAD occurs more commonly in white men than in black men. In women, the situation is reversed; black women develop CAD more commonly than white women do.

Other factors may also contribute to CAD. Hypertension, which occurs more commonly among black women of all ages and black men under age 45, increases the risk of CAD.

The not-so-golden years

Although serum cholesterol levels sometimes drop in older patients, age remains one of the most reliable indicators of CAD risk. As people age, the death rate from CAD increases steadily. Atherosclerosis becomes increasingly prevalent as men reach age 45 and women reach age 55.

Women and CAD

Although heart disease is the leading cause of death among women, diagnosis and treatment may not be as prompt as in men. Women share the same risk factors as men, but the clinical significance of those factors differs. With female patients, consider these facts:

• Female smokers have a risk of developing CAD that is two to six times greater than that of female nonsmokers.

• Hypertension is twice as common in women with heart disease as in men with the disease. A rise in systolic pressure of only 10 mm Hg can increase a woman's risk of ischemic heart disease and stroke by as much as 30%.

• The rate of heart disease in women increases after menopause, peaking at around age 70.

Weight and risk

• Being more than 30% overweight increases the likelihood that a woman will develop heart disease or stroke.

• The risk of CAD is greater for a woman carrying excess weight in the abdomen than it is for one carrying excess weight in the gluteal region.

• Gaining excess weight during adulthood may double the risk of CAD. In addition, weight fluctuation may have the same impact on CAD risk as obesity.

Other factors

• The risk of heart disease doubles when cholesterol levels exceed 200 mg/dl.

• Stress resulting from playing multiple roles in a family can increase a woman's (or man's) risk for developing CAD.

Modifiable risk factors

Although some risk factors can't be modified, such as age and gender, others can. (See *Controlling risk factors,* page 26.) Major modifiable risk factors include:

- cigarette smoking
- diabetes mellitus
- elevated homocystine levels
- elevated serum cholesterol levels
- elevated serum triglyceride levels
- high blood pressure.

High blood pressure = highest risk

Consistently high blood pressure — systolic or diastolic — poses the most important CAD risk. Because hypertension

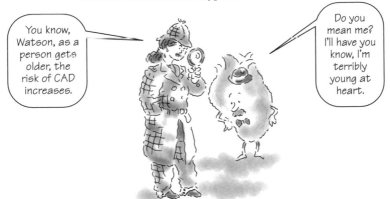

Advice from the experts

Controlling risk factors

To reduce the patient's risk of CAD, discuss ways of controlling certain risk factors, such as:
- alcohol restrictions
- caffeine-intake reduction
- diet low in fat and cholesterol
- exercise programs
- medical follow-up for such disorders as diabetes or hypertension
- programs to stop smoking
- stress-reduction techniques
- weight-reduction programs.

leads directly to atherosclerosis, the higher the blood pressure, the greater the chance of developing CAD. When combined with other risk factors, even a modest increase in blood pressure can lead to CAD.

> Why, the higher the blood pressure, the greater the risk.

> Tell me, how does blood pressure affect the risk of developing CAD?

Please put that out

Cigarette smoking puts patients at an extremely high risk for developing CAD. Smoking increases risk by:
• constricting blood vessels
• promoting thrombus formation
• lowering levels of vitamin C, necessary for cholesterol metabolism
• increasing catecholamine levels, which speeds the heart rate, increases blood pressure, and irritates arterial linings

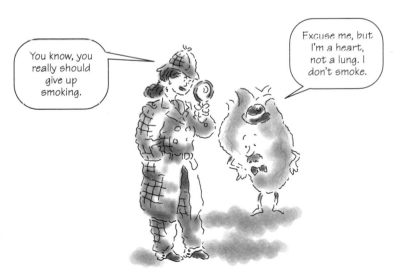

• stimulating platelet aggregation and the subsequent release of chemicals that cause vasospasm
• decreasing vital capacity
• decreasing cardiac output and promoting potentially fatal arrhythmias.

Filters don't lower risk

Contrary to what some patients believe, smoking filtered cigarettes doesn't reduce the risk of CAD. Smoking cigars or pipes may be less risky than cigarette smoking, but only slightly.

Cholesterol adds up

The risk of developing CAD increases when serum cholesterol levels are more than 200 mg/dl. Serum cholesterol levels of 200 mg/dl in a middle-aged adult indicates a relatively low risk of CAD. Levels of 200 to 240 mg/dl double the risk. About 27% of the U.S. population have cholesterol levels of 200 to 240 mg/dl.

Looking at low-density lipoproteins

Low-density lipoprotein (LDL) levels contribute to the formation of atherosclerotic plaques. Lipoproteins are complex molecules that transport lipids throughout the body. LDLs carry a high percentage of cholesterol and, at high blood levels, increase the production of atherosclerotic plaque. The normal LDL level is 62 to 185 mg/dl.

Hello to high-density lipoproteins

Another important lipoprotein, called high-density lipoprotein (HDL), consists mostly of protein and carries a lower percentage of cholesterol. Instead of increasing the production of atherosclerotic plaques, HDL removes lipids from cells. The normal HDL level is 29 to 77 mg/dl.

The good, the bad, and the aged

Increased LDL and decreased HDL levels substantially heighten the risk of CAD. Cholesterol levels as a whole tend to increase with age, declining only in the most advanced years.

Of A's, B's, and apolipoproteins

Apolipoprotein levels are also important determinants of CAD risk. Apolipoprotein A-1, the major protein component of HDL, is essential for the transport of cholesterol to the liver, so it can be excreted.

Hmmm, this patient has high LDL and low HDL levels. That means he's at increased risk for developing CAD.

Apolipoprotein B is the major protein component of LDL. A high ratio of A-1 to B indicates decreased risk of CAD.

Triglycerides are double trouble

Researchers believe that high serum triglyceride levels may increase the risk of CAD more than previously thought, especially if combined with low HDL levels. In the past, serum triglyceride levels below 500 mg/dl weren't considered cause for concern. Studies now indicate that levels exceeding 200 mg/dl actually double the risk of CAD.

Diabetes ups the ante, too.

The presence of diabetes consistently raises the risk of CAD. The risk of CAD in men with diabetes runs double that of men without diabetes. In women with diabetes, the risk is three times as great as in nondiabetic women. Researchers don't know why diabetes

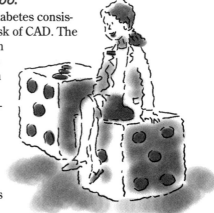

Diabetes significantly increases the odds of CAD.

predisposes a patient to CAD, but possible contributing factors include decreased HDL levels; high levels of glucose, which may cause glucose deposits on arterial walls; or increased platelet adhesion and other coagulation abnormalities.

Keep an eye on homocystine

High levels of the amino acid homocystine may also contribute to the development of CAD. Normal levels are 5 to 15 µmole. Recent studies show that folic acid (vitamin B_9) supplements can decrease the homocystine level, thus lowering CAD risk.

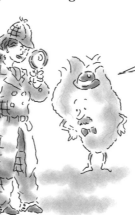

Don't forget the risk from homocystine.

Right-o. I shall be wise and B_9 myself forthwith.

Identifying contributing factors

Several factors can contribute to, but don't directly cause, the development of CAD. When combined with an assessment of known risk factors, contributing factors can help you identify patients at significant risk for CAD.

Consider a person at high risk for CAD if he possesses more than one major risk factor or one major risk factor combined with one or more of the following contributing factors:
- diet choices
- environmental factors
- gout
- left ventricular hypertrophy (LVH)
- obesity and lack of exercise
- oral contraceptive use
- stress.

No second helping of coffee or cake

A diet high in cholesterol and saturated fat may promote hypertension and raise blood cholesterol levels, thus increasing the risk of CAD. In addition, high caffeine intake may contribute to hypertension and arrhythmia.

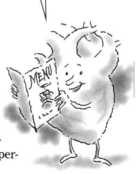

Make mine a low-cholesterol salad, with fat-free dressing, decaf coffee, and a small glass of wine.

Some studies show that moderate alcohol intake may reduce the risk of CAD and that excessive alcohol consumption damages the myocardium.

Another reason to move to Florida

High altitudes seem to reduce the incidence of CAD. Conversely, studies show higher CAD mortality rates among people living in predominantly cold, snowy regions. In addition, drinking water with a high mineral content seems to provide some protection against CAD, though this effect hasn't been attributed to a specific trace element.

Has gout gotcha?

Men with gout are twice as likely to develop CAD as men without gout. The higher risk may result from obesity, glucose intolerance, and increased blood lipids and blood pressure — all of which commonly occur with gout.

LVH causes the heart to pump harder

LVH occurs in nearly half of all patients who eventually die from cardiovascular disease, including CAD. LVH stems from chronic hypertension,

CAD from gout? Who'd a thunk it?

which forces the heart to pump harder against mounting pressure gradients.

Add the weight, increase the risk

Added body weight increases the risk of diabetes mellitus, hypertension, and elevated serum cholesterol levels, all of which contribute to CAD.

For people who don't exercise, inactivity seems to accompany decreased HDL levels, which increases the risk of developing CAD. Atherosclerosis also progresses more rapidly in inactive people, thus contributing to CAD development.

> Catch the exercise wave: Keep moving to cut CAD risk.

What the pill *doesn't* prevent

In most women, oral contraceptive use worsens the atherogenic process, causing plaques to develop more frequently. In particularly susceptible women, oral contraceptives also elevate blood pressure, another factor that can increase the likelihood of CAD. Women who smoke and use oral contraceptives place themselves at a particularly high risk for CAD and myocardial infarction (MI).

Stressed out

Stress hasn't been clinically proven to increase the risk of CAD but researchers know that, after a person develops CAD, the response to stress can lead to such further complications as MI. Scientists have also noted that a person with a tendency to react to stressful situations with anger or

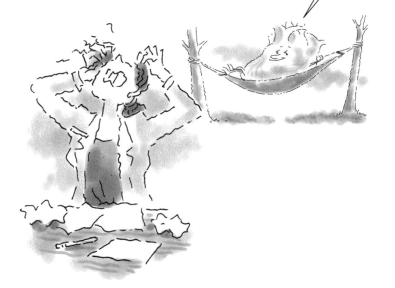

frustration may be more likely to develop CAD than one who reacts more calmly to stressful situations.

Preventing CAD progression

When a patient develops CAD, you can take steps to help prevent the disease from progressing. A program to limit the CAD progression should include steps to:
- reduce serum lipid levels
- change to a low-fat diet
- reduce stress
- reduce weight and participate in an exercise program
- stop smoking
- prevent or reduce hypertension
- control diabetes.

The more CAD progresses, the more the patient should limit fats.

Cutting cholesterol

Elevated cholesterol levels increase the risk that CAD will progress to MI or other serious complications. Patients can reduce their cholesterol levels through dietary changes and, when indicated, drug therapy.

Advice from the experts

Step I diet

The National Cholesterol Education Program recommends these criteria for the Step I diet for reducing the risk of developing CAD.

Food component	Amount
Total fat	less than 30%
Saturated fat	8% to 10%
Polyunsaturated fat	10% or less
Monounsaturated fat	up to 15%
Carbohydrates	50% to 60%
Protein	about 15%
Cholesterol	under 300 mg

Fighting fats

Diet modification follows a two-step approach, as recommended by the National Cholesterol Education Program. The Step I diet for adults with CAD includes restricting cholesterol intake and setting daily levels of fat, carbohydrates, and protein, according to percentages of the patient's total caloric intake. (See *Step I diet*.)

The Step II diet, for adults with significant heart disease, further restricts intake of saturated fat (less than 7%) and choles-

Advice from the experts

Cholesterol and the elderly

A recent study suggests that there is less of a link between cholesterol level and death from heart disease for older people than for patients in other age groups. For elderly patients with a history of heart disease, however, cholesterol still plays an important role.

When dealing with elderly patients with high cholesterol, consider the following facts:

• Reducing cholesterol by diet alone typically proves so difficult that few patients succeed at it.

• Patients with a history of MI and angina can reduce their chances of dying from heart disease by as much as 43% by lowering their cholesterol levels.

• Drug therapy for cholesterol reduction cuts the need for coronary artery bypass grafts by 34% and the occurrence of major coronary complications by 37%.

Effect of obesity

Obesity worsens the overall condition of elderly patients with high blood pressure or elevated total cholesterol. When an obese patient with hypertension loses weight, blood pressure and low-density lipoprotein levels drop. Weight reduction can be accomplished with regular exercise, decreased food intake, and a healthy diet.

terol (less than 200 mg). For elderly patients, a different dietary approach may be more appropriate. (See *Cholesterol and the elderly.*)

Breathe, relax, visualize

Implement techniques to reduce your patient's stress level. This includes discussing with the patient:
- sources of stress
- ways to minimize or eliminate stress
- strategies for coping with unavoidable stress
- relaxation techniques, such as deep breathing, progressive muscle relaxation, and visualization.

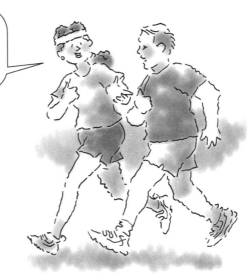

See? Jogging, walking, and other forms of aerobic exercise really can help improve your heart's performance.

Aerobic exercise — good...

Encourage regular exercise, and explore ways to incorporate exercise into the patient's daily routine. Walking and other aerobic exercises can improve oxygen extraction from the blood, even though they cause a slight increase in diastolic pressure. For patients with CAD, participation in an aerobic exercise program can:

- increase HDL levels
- decrease plasma catecholamines
- lower resting heart rate
- improve myocardial oxygenation, a benefit that may not decrease CAD risk but does fight complications.

> Can the patient exercise to slight breathlessness and still talk?

...anaerobic exercise — baaaad

Bear in mind that anaerobic (isometric) exercises can dramatically increase blood pressure. An elevated blood pressure may lead to angina, heart failure, or arrhythmia.

To assess a patient's exercise level, have him take the talk test. The talk test evaluates a patient's physical shape. Consider the patient in decent shape if he can exercise to the point of slight breathlessness and still talk without difficulty. He

should exercise to slight breathlessness
for 30 minutes at least 3 days each week.

Snuff out smoking

Nicotine is a vasoconstrictor that decreases arterial blood flow and causes endothelial injury. As a result, smoking can cause
or worsen CAD. To help the patient stop
smoking, discuss the:
• need to enroll in a smoking cessation
program
• location, cost, and other details of smoking cessation programs in the area
• possibility of using a nicotine transdermal system.

Hyperalert to hypertension

Help your patient with hypertension lower
his blood pressure. The following steps
can reduce blood pressure and help prevent CAD from worsening:
• reducing weight
• reducing stress
• exercising regularly
• maintaining blood pressure control
through regular checkups and follow-up
care.

Checked your blood sugar lately?

Patients with diabetes mellitus are at an increased risk for severe CAD. Be sure to discuss with the patient the importance of an early diagnosis and consistent control of blood glucose levels. Encourage regular checkups and follow-up care.

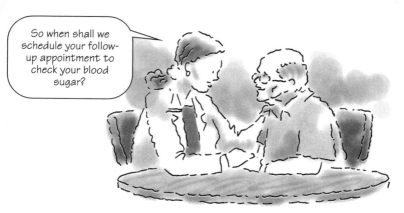

Quick quiz

1. Hypertension as a risk factor for CAD can be controlled through:
- A.   reducing weight.
- B.   taking iron supplements.
- C.   maintaining serum cholesterol above 200 mg/100 ml.

Answer: A. Hypertension can be managed through medication, weight reduction, stress reduction, and smoking cessation, all of which reduce a patient's risk of developing CAD.

2. The Step I diet includes an intake of monounsaturated fats of:
- A.   up to 15%.
- B.   up to 20%.
- C.   up to 30%.

Answer: A. The Step I diet recommends an intake of up to 15% monounsaturated fat.

3. In most women, contraceptive use tends to cause atherosclerotic plaques to form:
- A.   more frequently.
- B.   less frequently.
- C.   only in coronary arteries.

Answer: A. In most women, oral contraceptive use contributes to the atherogenic process, causing plaques to develop more frequently.

4. The risk of developing CAD increases when serum cholesterol levels are more than:
   A.   100 mg/dl.
   B.   200 mg/dl.
   C.   300 mg/dl.

Answer: B. The risk of developing CAD increases when serum cholesterol levels are more than 200 mg/dl.

Scoring

☆☆☆   If you answered all four questions correctly, right on! You're CAD Prevention Master!

☆☆   If you answered three questions correctly, good work! You're next in line for a CAD Prevention Attention Award!

☆   If you answered two or fewer questions correctly, fret not. Keep your sights set on winning the next Prevent-Athon for CAD.

3

Assessing patients with CAD

Key facts
- Assessing for cardiovascular risk factors can help identify CAD in its earliest stages.
- Angina is the hallmark symptom of CAD.
- Angina usually results from coronary atherosclerosis and may be a sign of CAD or it may indicate a worsening of the disease and the potential for myocardial infarction.

Taking a health history

A thorough history can help identify patients suffering from CAD and those at risk for developing CAD. Chest pain is usually the first overt sign of CAD. So, if a patient complains of chest pain, assume he's suffering a myocardial infarction (MI) until proven otherwise.

Evaluating the chief complaint

To determine the chief complaint, ask the patient why he's seeking medical care. If his chief complaint is chest pain or a related discomfort, ask:

• Where is the pain located?
• How would you describe it? Deep? Heavy? Squeezing? Aching? Burning?
• How severe is the pain?
• What, if anything, makes it worse? What makes it better?
• Does it cause shortness of breath?
• When did the pain start?
• How long have you had it?
• If it comes and goes, how long does it last?

• What were you doing when the pain started?

Also find out how his symptoms affect his daily routine and whether he has had any other associated symptoms.

Obtaining a history of angina

Angina pectoris, also known as chest pain, is the hallmark symptom of CAD. Angina results from an inadequate flow of oxygen to the myocardium. In angina, patients typically complain of pain in the anterior thoracic wall. (See *Angina road map,* page 48.)

Angina may be the first sign of CAD or a sign that CAD is progressing toward MI. (See *Blood flow and angina,* page 49.)

The many forms of angina

Angina usually appears in one of three forms: stable, unstable, or Prinzmetal's.

☝ Stable angina is predictable and lasts only a few minutes.

✌ Unstable angina, also called prein-farction angina, crescendo angina, acute coronary insufficiency, inter-mediate coronary syndrome, and im-

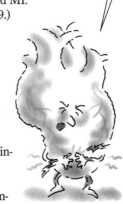

Oy, such a pain I've got. Angina is the hallmark symptom of CAD.

Angina road map

To obtain a more precise assessment of chest pain, ask the patient exactly where his pain is located. Angina usually occurs in the areas shown in this illustration.

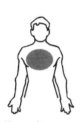

Upper chest

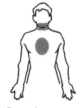

Beneath sternum, radiating to neck and jaw

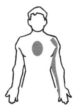

Beneath sternum, radiating down left arm

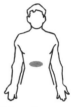

Epigastric area

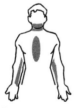

Epigastric area, radiating to neck, jaw, or arms

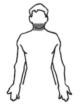

Neck and jaw

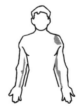

Left shoulder, inner aspect of both arms

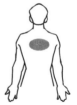

Intrascapular region

Now I get it!

Blood flow and angina

The heart receives oxygen-rich blood from the coronary arteries. At rest, the heart takes about 75% of the oxygen within the circulatory system, leaving 25% for the other organs.

As a result, the heart lacks oxygen reserve. Under stress, the heart must then rely on increased coronary blood flow to meet the added demands caused by the stress.

Pain of angina

The pain of angina arises from myocardial hypoxia. Causes of hypoxia include:

- decreased blood flow, resulting from atherosclerosis, thrombosis, embolism, or coronary artery spasm
- decreased oxygen-carrying capacity of the blood as in severe anemia
- increased myocardial workload, resulting from hypertension or aortic stenosis
- extracardial factors that increase the heart's workload and increase myocardial oxygen demand. (Possible extracardial factors include cocaine abuse, heavy exercise, or emotional stress.)

pending MI, is severe and frequently precedes an MI. (See *Identifying angina quickly,* pages 50 to 53.)

Prinzmetal's angina, also known as variant angina, occurs at rest, especially between midnight and 8 a.m.

(Text continues on page 52.)

Identifying angina quickly

This chart summarizes types of angina and the onset, duration, and course of each.

Type	Onset, course, and duration
Stable angina	• Predictable • Triggered by strenuous activity, cold weather, heightened emotional stress • Subtle at first, and then quickly reaching maximum intensity • Duration of a few seconds to 15 minutes
Unstable angina	• More severe than stable angina • Commonly preceding an MI • No triggers required • Duration of up to 30 minutes • Unpredictable course

Pain characteristics	Diagnosis
• Strangling sensation • Accompanied by anxiety • Pain commonly described as crushing, tightness, or heaviness • Pain usually located in substernal area with radiation to the left arm, jaw, neck, right arm, or back • Possibly accompanied by shortness of breath, diaphoresis, faintness, anxiety, or nausea • Typically relieved by rest or nitroglycerin tablets	• Based on patient's signs and symptoms and results of history and physical examination • Exercise stress test that shows ST-segment depression or down-sloping or horizontal depression of the ST segment • Holter monitor that shows ST-segment depression with certain activities even without complaints of chest pain • Exercise radionuclide angiography or coronary angiography, which helps confirm the diagnosis
• Pain resembling stable angina but more intense • Pain that may arouse patient from sleep • May occur with dyspnea, diaphoresis, nausea, or vomiting • Pain possibly radiating to previously uninvolved areas • Only partial relief provided by nitroglycerin; may require narcotics	• Electrocardiogram (ECG) showing transient changes in the ST segment • Patient's history and clinical condition, if no ECG changes

Identifying angina quickly *(continued)*

Type	Onset, course, and duration
Prinzmetal's, or variant, angina	• Occurring at rest • Resulting from coronary artery spasm • Not produced by exertion or stress • Possible without coronary atherosclerosis • Frequently no risk factors for CAD present • Affecting some heavy smokers • Typical occurrence at the same time each day • Frequent occurrences between midnight and 8 a.m. • Possibly accompanied by stable angina

In addition, you may encounter three rare forms of angina. Nocturnal angina occurs at night while the patient is lying down. Intractable angina, also known as refractory angina, involves severe, incapacitating anginal pain. The third form, silent ischemia, is considered a form of angina even though the patient remains asymptomatic. Objective evidence of this form of angina generally comes from results of a stress test or Holter (long-term) monitoring.

Pain characteristics	Diagnosis
• Similar to unstable angina • Sudden pain located in the substernal chest • Pain ranging from a feeling of heaviness to a crushing discomfort • Possibly accompanied by shortness of breath, diaphoresis, nausea, or vomiting • Prompt relief from nitroglycerin	• ECG that shows marked ST-segment elevation during chest pain that quickly disappears with nitroglycerin or other pain control measures • Coronary angiography possibly indicated for a patient with suspected coronary artery spasm

Keep in mind that angina can be caused by lots of conditions.

Causes of angina

Angina may be precipitated by a number of factors, including:
- cold temperatures
- strong emotions, such as fright or anger
- exercise, including walking after a large meal or walking against the wind
- raising arms above the head
- sexual activity.

Angina mimics

Although angina is commonly caused by CAD, angina-like pain can stem from a variety of sources. Those sources include:

- acute bronchitis
- anxiety
- aortic aneurysm
- cholecystitis
- esophagitis
- lung abscess
- musculoskeletal strain
- MI
- pancreatitis
- peptic ulcer
- pneumonia
- pneumothorax
- pulmonary embolism
- rib fracture
- tuberculosis
- withdrawal from beta blockers.

Of course, not all chest pain indicates a cardiac condition. When assessing the patient, ask questions designed to differentiate cardiac from noncardiac pain. (See *Asking the right questions.*)

Asking the right questions

The following questions can help you distinguish cardiac from non-cardiac pain. Ask the patient:

Does the discomfort change or worsen when you shift position? (Angina isn't affected by body position changes.)

Does a deep breath make the discomfort better or worse? (Angina isn't aggravated by respirations.)

Can you point to the discomfort with one finger? (Angina tends to be diffuse, not sharply localized.)

Does the discomfort seem like it comes from deep within or close to the surface? (Angina typically feels like it comes from deep within.)

Does the discomfort seem intense, sharp, dull, or knifelike? (Angina is typically described as a dull ache, seldom sharp or stabbing.)

Exploring medical history

Ask the patient about a history of:
• major acute or chronic illnesses requiring hospitalization
• prescription, over-the-counter, or recreational drug use

- allergies to food, drugs, herbal medicine, or other agents
- cardiovascular risk factors.

Gettin' to know the family

Family history can play a large role in a patient's susceptibility to CAD. Ask questions about blood relatives with:

- diabetes mellitus
- heart disease
- hypertension
- kidney disease
- stroke.

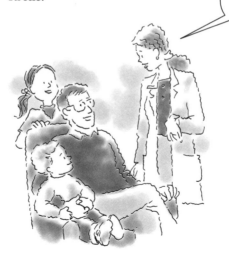

Family history is important. Do you have any relatives with heart disease or high blood pressure?

Gettin' to know the patient

When taking a patient's social history, pay particular attention to smoking, signs of stress, exercise habits, and other factors that place a patient at risk for CAD. Ask questions about:
- alcohol use
- daily activities
- diet
- educational background
- exercise habits
- living arrangements

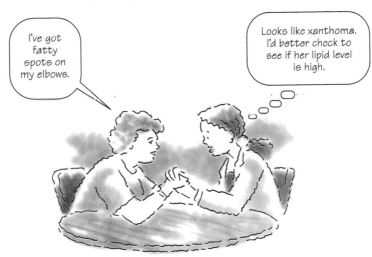

- occupation
- sleep habits
- smoking.

Examining a patient with CAD

A thorough physical examination can help determine the presence of atherosclerotic disease. To examine a patient who has CAD or whom you suspect may have it, inspect first and then percuss, palpate, and auscultate.

Inspection

A thorough inspection may reveal evidence of atherosclerotic disease, such as:
- cyanosis
- increased light reflexes and arteriovenous nicking on ophthalmic examination, which may suggest hypertension
- peripheral edema
- skin color changes
- xanthelasma (yellow, fatty deposits located on the eyelids that suggest elevated serum cholesterol levels)
- xanthoma (yellow, fatty deposits on the skin — such as at the elbows — that suggest elevated lipid levels).

Palpation

After inspecting the patient's skin, palpate the chest and neck to detect abnormal pulsations or superficial abnormalities that may indicate CAD. Palpation may reveal:

• abnormal contraction of the cardiac impulse, such as left ventricular akinesia or dyskinesia

• masses, tenderness, or other superficial abnormalities of the neck or chest

• subcutaneous emphysema, which feels as if the tissue beneath the skin is popping

• tracheal deviation.

Percussion

Although not as useful as other methods of assessment for a cardiovascular examination, percussion may help you locate cardiac borders and determine heart size. Begin percussing at the anterior axillary line and percuss toward the sternum along the fifth intercostal space.

Once resonant, now dull

The sound changes from resonance to dullness at the left border of the heart, nor-

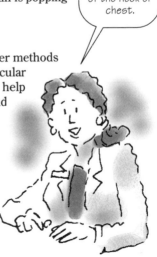

Palpation may reveal a number of superficial abnormalities of the neck or chest.

mally at the midclavicular line. The right border is usually aligned with the sternum and can't be percussed.

Auscultation

You can learn a great deal about the heart through auscultation. Cardiac auscultation requires a methodical approach and lots and lots of practice. Take your time, and concentrate hard when auscultating.

Abnormalities that speak to you

When auscultating the chest for abnormalities, check for the presence of:
• bruits, especially along the carotid arteries
• S_3 heart sound
• S_4 heart sound or late systolic murmur.

Also check the rate and depth of respirations to detect respiratory problems and blood pressure to detect hypertension.

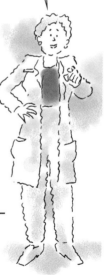

How do you get to Auscultation Hall? Practice, practice, practice.

Diagnostic tests

A number of laboratory tests can be used to identify patients at risk for

CAD as well to confirm CAD's development.

Lipid profile

A lipid profile test that reveals high levels of low-density lipoproteins may indicate atherosclerosis. High levels of high-density lipoproteins (above 75 mg/dl), however, may indicate that the patient is at lower risk for developing CAD. Consider a serum cholesterol level above 200 mg/dl as a CAD risk factor.

Apolipoprotein tests also provide evidence of CAD risk. Increased levels of apolipoprotein B indicate high risk of CAD.

Isoenzymes

A cardiac isoenzyme test, which measures enzyme levels of heart muscle cells, can indicate if CAD has caused injury to myocardial tissues. In myocardial ischemia, breaks in myocardial cell membranes lead to the release of certain isoenzymes into the bloodstream. The timing and extent of increases and decreases in serum levels of these enzymes provide a measurement of cardiac damage.

Is the serum cholesterol over 200 mg/dl? Then the patient has an increased risk of developing CAD.

Complete blood count

A complete blood count provides indirect evidence of myocardial workload. The hematocrit (HCT) is a percentage of the volume of red blood cells (RBCs) in a sample of whole blood, providing a measurement of viscosity.

The more red blood cells are contained in the blood, the more viscous the blood is. The more viscous the blood, the greater the peripheral vascular resistance and, as a result, the greater the cardiac workload.

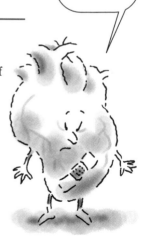

Help! I'm injured. Better measure my isoenzyme levels to see how badly.

Diagnostic procedures

Several procedures may be performed to confirm the presence of CAD, including an electrocardiogram (ECG), a treadmill or bicycle exercise stress test, coronary angiography, rapid atrial pacing, and myocardial perfusion imaging.

ECG

A 12-lead ECG, performed when the patient is experiencing chest pain, can identify areas of decreased blood supply. It can also identify arrhythmias such as premature ventricular contractions. During pain-free periods, an ECG may show normal results, depending on the extent of myocardial damage.

Exercise stress test

In this procedure, the patient's heart is monitored by ECG while he exercises at a controlled rate on a treadmill or bicycle. As the heart beats faster, the ECG may reveal evidence of myocardial ischemia.

If exercise prompts pain...

If CAD has developed, chest pain may occur as the patient's heart rate and myocardial oxygen demand increase. The test is considered positive if it shows ST-segment depression of 1 mm, 0.08 second after the J point (where the QRS complex ends and the ST segment begins).

If the patient is unable to exercise, drugs may be used to mimic exercise by increasing

> Placing stress on the heart during an exercise test may reveal evidence of myocardial ischemia.

the patient's heart rate and cardiac work-load.

How it works

In an exercise stress test, expect the following steps to occur:

• Chest electrodes are placed according to the cardiac lead system selected and secured with tape or a rubber belt. Lead wires are connected to the chest electrodes.

• A stable baseline tracing is made and checked for arrhythmia. Check the patient's blood pressure, and auscultate his chest for crackles or an S_3 or S_4 heart sound.

• The patient is shown how to use the treadmill or bicycle. In a treadmill test, the treadmill speed is gradually increased. In a bicycle test, the patient is told to pedal until he reaches the desired speed, as shown on the speedometer.

• During either test, monitor the patient for blood pressure or ECG changes. Tell the patient to report dizziness, light-headedness, leg fatigue, dyspnea, or chest pain. Observe for diaphoresis or pallor. The test is stopped if signs or symptoms become severe.

• Testing typically stops when the patient reaches the target heart rate. Activity is then stopped gradually to provide a cooldown.

• After exercising, the patient is asked to sit for 10 to 15 minutes or until his ECG returns to baseline. His blood pressure and ECG are monitored throughout the cooldown.

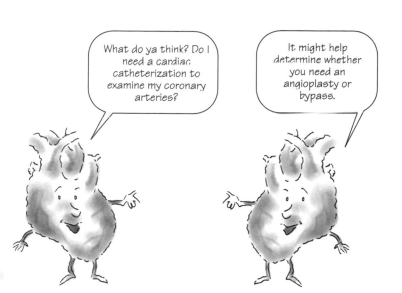

What do ya think? Do I need a cardiac catheterization to examine my coronary arteries?

It might help determine whether you need an angioplasty or bypass.

Cardiac catheterization

This procedure, also known as coronary angiography, is performed to visualize the coronary arteries. It evaluates the need for coronary angioplasty or bypass surgery and can reveal the location and extent of:

• artery condition distal to a narrowing
• collateral circulation
• coronary artery stenosis
• arterial obstruction.

How it works: Before

A number of tasks must be completed prior to a cardiac catheterization. Before the test, explain to the patient that he:

• will be asked to lie completely still on a table that tilts
• will have an I.V. inserted
• will have his heart beat and vital signs monitored
• may feel flushed following the injection if a contrast medium is used, but that the feeling should pass
• may be asked to cough during the test
• should take nothing by mouth for 6 to 8 hours before the test.

In addition, before the test, you should:
• ask the patient about allergies to shellfish, iodine, or contrast medium
• instruct the patient to void before the test
• prepare the area where the catheter will be inserted, as ordered
• remove the patient's jewelry and dentures
• record the patient's vital signs
• mark the location of pedal pulses
• medicate the patient as ordered
• discuss the informed consent form with the patient.

How it works: During

A cardiac catheterization usually takes ½ hour to 1 hour. During the test, expect the following steps:

A nurse threads a catheter into the patient's artery or vein (usually the brachial artery or vein or the femoral artery or vein), depending on side of the heart to be evaluated.

The patient receives a local anesthetic.

A doctor threads a catheter into the patient's heart and evaluates pressure readings and oxygen saturation.

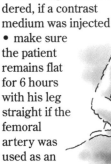 The doctors injects a contrast medium to show heart chambers and structures under fluoroscopy and assess the coronary arteries for signs of CAD.

How it works: After

When the cardiac catheterization is finished, you should:
• monitor the patient's vital signs and peripheral pulses, as ordered
• monitor the catheter insertion site for bleeding or hematoma
• use a pressure dressing and sandbag over the insertion site, as ordered
• encourage fluids, as ordered, if a contrast medium was injected
• make sure the patient remains flat for 6 hours with his leg straight if the femoral artery was used as an insertion site

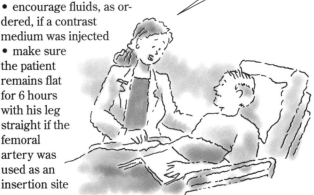

Because we used an artery in your groin for your cardiac catheterization, you'll need to lie flat with your leg straight for 6 hours.

• make sure the patient keeps his arm immobile for 3 hours, if the brachial vein was used as an insertion site.

Rapid atrial pacing

Rapid atrial pacing can be used instead of an exercise test to diagnose angina. This test allows the doctor to investigate left ventricular function without prompting changes in cardiac output, afterload, or circulating catecholamines.

Myocardial perfusion imaging

Myocardial perfusion imaging, a noninvasive study, uses thallium or technetium to identify ischemic areas of the myocardium. These areas show up as "cold spots" on the scan, meaning that the color of these areas differs from surrounding areas. This procedure is commonly used in conjunction with a treadmill exercise stress test.

Quick quiz

1. Common types of angina include:
   A. intractable angina.
   B. Prinzmetal's angina.
   C. silent ischemia.

Answer: B. Prinzmetal's angina, along with stable and unstable angina, are the most common types of angina.

2. Xanthelasma noted on the eyelids is a physical finding that suggests:
   A. decreased red blood cell count.
   B. elevated blood lipid levels.
   C. elevated cardiac isoenzyme levels.

Answer: B. Xanthelasma are yellow, fatty deposits located on the eyelids that suggest elevated blood lipid levels.

3. When percussing the chest, the sound at the left border of the heart changes from:
   A. dullness to resonance.
   B. hyperresonance to resonance.
   C. resonance to dullness.

Answer: C. The sound changes from resonance to dullness at the left border of the heart, normally at the midclavicular line.

4. For the first 6 hours after a patient's cardiac catheterization in which the femoral artery is used, you should make sure the patient:

    A. remains flat in bed.

    B. walks at least a few feet.

    C. performs range-of-motion exercises with the affected limb.

Answer: A. The patient who has had a femoral artery insertion site used for cardiac catheterization should remain flat in bed for 6 hours.

5. The most common noninvasive test for detecting CAD is:

    A. an exercise stress test.

    B. coronary angiography.

    C. serial ECG readings.

Answer: A. An exercise stress test is the most common noninvasive method to detect CAD.

Scoring

☆☆☆ If you answered all five questions correctly, super! You're the Stress Test Champ!

☆☆ If you answered four questions correctly, hooray! Your diagnostic skills have earned you a Prinzmetal medal.

☆ If you answered three or fewer questions correctly, it's OK. You're neither intractable nor unstable. With practice, you might be our next Mighty Myocardial Master!

4

Treating patients with CAD

Key facts

♦ Noninvasive measures to treat CAD include drug therapy (usually with aspirin, antilipemics, beta blockers, calcium channel blockers, or nitrates) and cardiac rehabilitation.

♦ Percutaneous transluminal coronary angioplasty is a nonsurgical alternative to bypass surgery that improves coronary blood flow.

♦ Coronary artery bypass grafting restores blood flow to the heart by bypassing a blockage in a coronary artery.

♦ By participating in a rehabilitation program, a patient with CAD can maintain fitness and reduce the risk of another cardiac event.

Treating CAD

Treatment for CAD has seven goals: alleviating pain, increasing the oxygen supply, reducing myocardial oxygen demand, improving coronary artery perfusion, lessening myocardial workload, preventing myocardial infarction (MI), and preventing unstable angina.

Type of treatment

CAD can be treated using noninvasive or invasive methods. The type of treatment that a patient receives depends on four main factors:

- frequency of the patient's angina
- duration of the angina
- severity of the angina
- hemodynamic changes, such as changes in blood pressure, heart rate, or cardiac output.

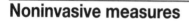

> Treatment for CAD can be invasive or noninvasive, depending on several factors.

Noninvasive measures

Noninvasive methods can be used to increase myocardial oxygen supply, decrease myocardial oxygen demand, and improve coronary artery perfusion. These methods include:

- bed rest (immediately following an acute episode)
- drug therapy
- supplemental oxygen.

Bed rest

Bed rest decreases demands on the heart, thereby lessening the myocardial

Noninvasive measures
• Bed rest
• Drug therapy
• Supplemental oxygen

workload and oxygen demand. It may also promote relaxation and decrease anxiety, thereby keeping the heart rate down and decreasing cardiac workload. Generally, a patient with CAD is kept on bed rest for not more than 24 hours before starting on a regimen of gradually increasing exercise.

Drug therapy

Several different types of drugs can be used to reduce the severity of CAD or risk of complications. (See *Drug therapy*, pages 76 to 85.)

Supplemental oxygen

Supplemental oxygen decreases the patient's myocardial workload and increases the patient's oxygen level. As a result, myocardial tissues can receive adequate amounts of oxygen.

(Text continues on page 85.)

Drug therapy

A patient with CAD can be treated with a variety of medications, including antilipemics, beta blockers, calcium channel blockers, and nitrates. This table highlights adverse reactions and special considerations for drugs used to treat a patient with CAD.

Antilipemics

Antilipemics reduce serum cholesterol levels by decreasing lipoprotein synthesis or by increasing lipoprotein catabolism (breakdown). Lowering blood levels of lipids to normal reduces myocardial workload. Commonly prescribed antilipemics include cholestyramine, colestipol hydrochloride, fluvastatin sodium, gemfibrozil, lovastatin, pravastatin sodium, and simvastatin.

cholestyramine
Trade name: Questran

Adverse reactions
Adverse reactions include constipation, abdominal discomfort, nausea, rash, and vitamin A, D, and K deficiency.

Special considerations
• Monitor bowel habits. Encourage the patient to follow a diet high in fiber and fluids.
• Instruct the patient never to take drug in its dry form; esophageal irritation or severe constipation may result
• Sprinkle powder on surface of a large glass containing the patient's preferred beverage. Let stand a few minutes, then stir. After drinking, add a small amount of liquid to the same glass, swirl, and have patient drink to ensure ingestion of entire dose.
• Use cautiously in patients predisposed to constipation.

Drug therapy *(continued)*

colestipol hydrochloride
Trade name: Colestid

Adverse reactions
Adverse reactions include headache, constipation, nausea, vomiting, rash, irritation of tongue and perianal area, and vitamin A, D, E, and K deficiency.

Special considerations
• Monitor bowel habits, serum cholesterol levels, and triglyceride levels.
• Instruct the patient never to take drug in its dry form.
• To enhance palatability, mix and refrigerate the next day's dose the previous evening.
• Use cautiously in patients predisposed to constipation.

fluvastatin sodium
Trade name: Lescol

Adverse reactions
Adverse reactions include dyspepsia, diarrhea, hemolytic anemia, sinusitis, muscle pain, and hypersensitivity reactions.

Special considerations
• Watch for signs of myositis.
• Use cautiously in patients with severe renal impairment, history of liver disease, or in patients who are heavy drinkers.

gemfibrozil
Trade name: Lopid

Adverse reactions
Adverse reactions include blurred vision, headache, dizziness, abdominal and epigastric pain, diarrhea, nausea, anemia, bile duct obstruction, elevated liver enzymes, rash, and painful extremities.

(continued)

Drug therapy *(continued)*

gemfibrozil *(continued)*

Special considerations
- Monitor complete blood count and liver function tests.
- Instruct patient to take drug 30 minutes before breakfast and dinner.
- Advise the patient to report steatorrhea or other signs of bile duct obstruction.

lovastatin
Trade name: Mevacor

Adverse reactions
Adverse reactions include headache, dizziness, peripheral neuropathy, blurred vision, constipation, diarrhea, dyspepsia, abdominal pain or cramps, rash, muscle cramps, myalgia, and abnormal liver test results.

Special considerations
• Encourage the patient to follow a low-fat diet and to take medication with evening meal.
• Use cautiously in patients who are heavy drinkers.

pravastatin sodium
Trade name: Pravachol

Adverse reactions
Adverse reactions include headache, dizziness, vomiting, nausea, diarrhea, cough, and muscle pain.

Special considerations
• Encourage the patient to follow a low-fat diet and to take medication with evening meal.
• Use cautiously in patients who are heavy drinkers.

Drug therapy *(continued)*

simvastatin
Trade name: Zocor

Adverse reactions
Adverse reactions include headache, asthenia, abdominal pain, constipation, diarrhea, nausea, vomiting, and elevated liver enzymes.

Special considerations
• Encourage the patient to follow a low-fat diet and to take medication with evening meal.
• Use cautiously in patients who are heavy drinkers.

Beta-adrenergic blockers

Beta-adrenergic blockers, more commonly called beta blockers, alleviate anginal symptoms by blocking catecholamine stimulation of beta-adrenergic receptors. Beta$_1$-adrenergic receptors are located in the bronchioles and arterial smooth muscles. The sympathetic nervous system sends signals to the beta$_1$ receptors, which tell the heart how fast to beat.

Beta blockers stop those signals. This blockage reduces myocardial response, which leads to lower blood pressure and reduced myocardial oxygen demand. Commonly ordered beta blockers include nadolol and propranolol hydrochloride.

nadolol
Trade name: Corgard

Adverse reactions
Adverse reactions include fatigue, lethargy, bradycardia, hypotension, heart failure, nausea, vomiting, diarrhea, rash, fever, and increased airway resistance.

(continued)

Drug therapy *(continued)*

nadolol *(continued)*

Special considerations
• Always check the patient's apical pulse before giving drug. If it's slower than 60 beats/minute, withhold the drug and notify the primary care provider.
• Monitor blood pressure frequently. If severe hypotension develops, administer a vasopressor, as prescribed.
• Dosage should be reduced gradually over 1 to 2 weeks.
• Caution patients not to suddenly discontinue drug; doing so can exacerbate angina or myocardial infarction (MI).
• Use cautiously in patients with a history of heart failure, chronic bronchitis, emphysema, or diabetes.
• Be aware that nadolol masks common signs of shock and hyperthyroidism.

propranolol hydrochloride
Trade name: Inderal

Adverse reactions
Adverse reactions include fatigue, lethargy, vivid dreams, mental depression, bradycardia, hypotension, heart failure, intermittent claudication, nausea, vomiting, diarrhea, increased airway resistance, rash, fever, and arthralgia.

Special considerations
• Use cautiously in patients with diabetes, renal impairment, hepatic disease, and nonallergic bronchospastic disease and in patients taking other antihypertensives.
• Administer with meals.
• Monitor blood pressure frequently. If severe hypotension develops, notify the doctor.
• Don't discontinue the drug suddenly; doing so can exacerbate angina or MI.

Drug therapy *(continued)*

Calcium channel blockers

Calcium channel blockers prevent the passage of calcium ions across the myocardial cell membrane, which results in vasodilation of coronary and peripheral arteries, decreased contractile force of the myocardium, and decreased cardiac workload. Coronary blood flow is increased, and myocardial oxygen demand is decreased. Commonly prescribed calcium channel blockers include bepridil hydrochloride, diltiazem hydrochloride, nifedipine, and verapamil.

bepridil hydrochloride
Trade name: Vascor

Adverse reactions
Adverse reactions include dizziness, edema, flushing, palpitations, ventricular arrhythmia, nausea, diarrhea, agranulocytosis, rash, and dyspnea.

Special considerations
• Because the drug prolongs the QT interval, monitor the patient's electrocardiogram (ECG) for ventricular arrhythmia.
• Tell the patient to report unusual bruising or bleeding or signs of infection.
• Use cautiously in patients with left bundle branch block, sinus bradycardia, impaired renal or hepatic function, or heart failure.

diltiazem hydrochloride
Trade name: Cardizem

Adverse reactions
Adverse reactions include headache, fatigue, drowsiness, insomnia, edema, arrhythmia, bradycardia, hypotension, heart failure, nausea, vomiting, diarrhea, nocturia, polyuria, rash, pruritus, and photosensitivity.

(continued)

Drug therapy *(continued)*

diltiazem hydrochloride

Special considerations
- Assist the patient with ambulation during initiation of therapy.
- Use cautiously in elderly patients; the drug's duration of action may be prolonged.
- If systolic blood pressure is below 90 mm Hg or the heart rate is below 60 beats/minute, withhold the dose and notify the primary care provider.

nifedipine
Trade name: Procardia

Adverse reactions
Adverse reactions include dizziness, light-headedness, flushing, headache, weakness, hypotension, palpitations, peripheral edema, nasal congestion, nausea, heartburn, diarrhea, dyspnea, muscle cramps, and hypokalemia.

Special considerations
- Monitor blood pressure and serum potassium levels.
- Continuous blood pressure and ECG monitoring are recommended.
- When rapid response to the drug is desired, instruct the patient to bite and then swallow the capsule.
- Use cautiously in patients with heart failure or hypotension and in the elderly.

verapamil hydrochloride
Trade name: Calan, Isoptin

Adverse reactions
Adverse reactions include dizziness, headache, fatigue, transient hypotension, bradycardia, heart failure, peripheral edema, constipation, nausea, and elevated liver enzymes.

Drug therapy *(continued)*

verapamil hydrochloride *(continued)*

Special considerations
- Advise the patient to take the drug with food.
- Because dizziness may occur, assist the patient with ambulation.

Special considerations
- Use cautiously in patients with increased intracranial pressure, hepatic disease, or renal disease, and in the elderly.
- To minimize the risk of adverse reactions, give I.V. doses over at least 3 minutes.
- Place patient on a cardiac monitor and pay special attention to R-R intervals during therapy.

Nitrates

Nitrates relax smooth muscles throughout the body, including the vascular system. This relaxation decreases myocardial workload and oxygen demand. Commonly prescribed nitrates include isosorbide dinitrate and nitroglycerin.

isosorbide dinitrate
Trade name: Isorbid, Isordil, Sorbitrate

Adverse reactions
Adverse reactions include headache, dizziness, weakness, orthostatic hypotension, tachycardia, ankle edema, nausea, vomiting, flushing, and sublingual burning.

Special considerations
- Advise the patient to take sublingual tablet at the first sign of attack.
- To prevent development of tolerance, a nitrate-free interval of 8 to 12 hours a day is recommended.
- Know that hypotensive effects are possible if used with an antihypertensive.

(continued)

Drug therapy *(continued)*

nitroglycerin

Trade name: Nitro-Bid, Nitro-Dur, Nitrostat, Transderm-Nitro, Tridil

Adverse reactions

Adverse reactions include headache, dizziness, weakness, orthostatic hypotension, tachycardia, flushing, palpitations, nausea, vomiting, contact dermatitis, and sublingual burning.

Special considerations

I.V. use

• Administer with an infusion control device, and titrate to desired response.

• Mix in glass bottles. Avoid using I.V. filters; the drug binds to plastic. Also use special nonabsorbent (non-PVC) tubing.

• Closely monitor vital signs during the infusion.

• When changing the concentration of nitroglycerin infusion, flush the I.V. administration set with 15 to 20 ml of the new concentration before use.

Oral

• Advise the patient to take the drug on an empty stomach, either 30 minutes before or 1 to 2 hours after a meal.

• Tell the patient not to chew the tablet.

Sublingual

• Instruct the patient to take the drug at the first sign of pain. The dose may be repeated every 5 minutes to a maximum of 3 doses. If the patient doesn't experience relief, advise him to seek medical help immediately.

Buccal

• Instruct the patient to place the tablet between the lip and gum above the incisors, or between the cheek and gum.

Aerosol

• Tell the patient to spray one dose under the tongue, and then to close his mouth.

• Instruct the patient not to inhale the spray or swallow the spray immediately.

Drug therapy *(continued)*

nitroglycerin *(continued)*
• Tell the patient the dose may be repeated in 3 to 5 minutes, not to exceed 3 doses in 15 minutes.
• Advise the patient to use the drug before performing a strenuous job and to sit down after use.
Patch
• To apply, Remove the backing of the patch and apply the patch to any nonhairy area except the distal parts of the arms or legs.
• Remember to remove the old patch before applying a new one.

Invasive measures

If drug therapy and other noninvasive measures don't lower or eliminate the patient's angina, an invasive measure may be required. The most commonly used invasive measures for treating CAD include percutaneous transluminal coronary angioplasty (PTCA) and coronary artery bypass graft (CABG).

PTCA

PTCA, a nonsurgical alternative to bypass surgery, is used to improve blood flow through the coronary arteries. During a PTCA, a balloon-tipped catheter

is placed in a stenosed coronary artery.
(See *What happens in PTCA,* page 89.)
Inflation of the balloon widens the vessel
lumen by compressing the plaque.

Step-by-step PTCA

In a PTCA, a doctor guides a catheter
through the ascending aorta. The
catheter is then passed into the ostium
(opening) of either the right or left coronary artery. An angiogram is then performed.

Then the doctor inserts a dilating
catheter through the guiding catheter
and into the artery's stenotic area. The
catheter allows for continuous blood
pressure monitoring, which helps
locate blockages within the coronary artery. The catheter measures the pressure gradient prior
to the lesion and within the lesion.

When the lesion has been as-
sessed, the doctor inflates the
balloon on the catheter for 30 to
60 seconds, using a mixture of
contrast medium and saline
solution in equal proportions.
Balloon inflation is controlled with a

> PTCA can
> improve
> blood flow
> through my
> arteries
> and widen
> my vessel
> lumen.
> Hooray!

Now I get it!

What happens in PTCA

During a percutaneous transluminal coronary angioplasty (PTCA), a balloon-tipped catheter is placed into a stenosed coronary artery. Inflation of the balloon widens the vessel lumen by compressing the plaque.

Compression of the plaque triggers platelet aggregation and the release of a potent vasodilator called prostacyclin from the vessel wall, thereby stretching the walls of the coronary arteries even more.

pressure pump set between 3 and 6.5 atmospheres. Another angiogram is performed to evaluate the angioplasty's effect.

Stent placement

Placement of an intracoronary stent during a PTCA may decrease the risk of restenosis, a possible complication of PTCA. A stent is a metallic device with variations of a honeycomb configuration. The stent and an inflatable balloon are inserted into the stenosed artery. When the balloon is inflated, the stent is expanded. After the balloon is deflated, the stent remains in place.

Preventive cracks

Balloon inflation produces cracks of various depths in the plaque. These cracks may provide additional channels for blood flow through the coronary arteries and possibly help prevent early restenosis of the vessel after angioplasty.

PTCA perks

Compared with CABG, a more invasive procedure, PTCA offers these benefits:

• Hospitalization lasts only 1 to 2 days.

• The patient is usually up and walking within a day.

• In many instances, the patient can return to work in just a few weeks.

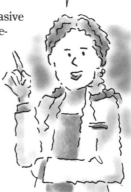

Balloon inflation lasts from 30 to 60 seconds and is tightly controlled by a pressure pump.

Before a PTCA

When caring for a patient about to undergo a PTCA, make sure to:

• assess the cardiovascular system.

• maintain telemetry monitoring.

- look for signs of cardiac arrhythmia, such as ventricular tachycardia or premature ventricular contractions
- assess the patient's knowledge of the procedure. If necessary, teach the patient about the procedure. Review the risks and possible complications.
- remind the patient of the importance of remaining awake and assisting with the proper placement of the catheter by taking deep breaths when instructed.
- tell the patient that CABG may be necessary if PTCA fails.

During a PTCA

If you are assisting during PTCA, expect to perform the following care measures:
- assess the patient for complications
- monitor hemodynamic status
- maintain telemetry monitoring and observe for signs of arrhythmia
- monitor for bleeding at the puncture site
- monitor for chest pain
- track cardiac enzyme levels
- measure intake and output.

Complications of PTCA
• Coronary artery occlusion
• Coronary artery spasm
• Dissection of the coronary artery
• Hematoma
• Hemorrhage
• MI
• Restenosis
• Rupture

After a PTCA

After a PTCA has been completed, perform the following tasks:
• assess for complications
• monitor hemodynamic status, making sure to use the arterial sheath for pressure measurements
• maintain telemetry monitoring and observe for signs of arrhythmia
• monitor for bleeding at the puncture site
• track cardiac enzyme levels
• apply a pressure dressing after sheath removal

- assess circulation
- monitor for chest pain, shortness of breath, and changes in mental status
- remind the patient about the importance of taking prescribed drugs properly and monitoring risk factors.

CABG

CABG restores blood flow to an ischemic heart by bypassing the blockage in the coronary artery. If successful, CABG improves blood supply, relieves symptoms, and extends the patient's life.

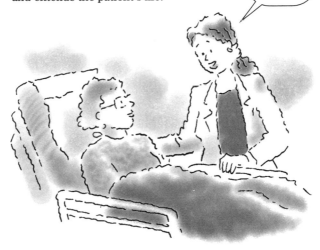

Because three of your arteries are blocked, the doctor will perform a bypass graft.

CABG may be performed on patients with:

• anatomy unsuitable for angioplasty

• chronic disabling angina pectoris unresponsive to medical therapy

• continuing angina pectoris after MI

• history of failed angioplasty

• stenosis of the left main coronary artery, in which the artery narrows by more than half its diameter

• three or more vessels involved

• unstable or preinfarction angina unresponsive to medical therapy.

What happens

Here's what happens during a CABG:

• The surgical team prepares the patient for cardiopulmonary bypass.

• The surgeon excises a saphenous vein graft from the leg.

• The surgeon cannulates the right atrium to divert blood to the heart-lung machine. (See *Understanding the heart-lung machine.*)

• Oxygenated blood returns from the heart-lung machine to the arterial system through an arterial cannula positioned in the ascending aortic arch.

Now I get it!

Understanding the heart-lung machine

A heart-lung machine circulates blood during coronary artery bypass surgery. The machine consists of three main parts: a pump, an oxygenator with a reservoir, and plastic circuitry.

Large tubes divert blood away from the right atrium (or from the right vena cava), as shown below. Venous blood drains into a reservoir positioned lower than the patient's right atrium. A second, smaller reservoir collects blood from the operative field.

Minimizing clotting

Both reservoirs contain filters to minimize clotting. After oxygenation, filtration, dilution, and temperature alterations, the blood returns to the patient through a tube in the ascending aorta or femoral artery.

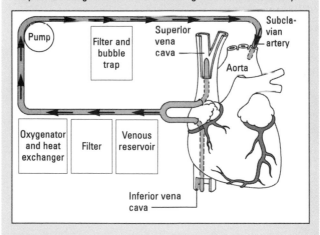

• To prevent clotting, the patient's blood is diluted and heparinized.

• To conserve oxygen, the patient's body temperature is reduced to 68° to 82.4° F (20° to 28° C).

• The surgeon injects a cold cardio-plegic solution into the heart and then sews the grafts into place. The graft is joined proximally to the ascending aorta and distally to the coronary arteries, beyond the occlusion site. The left internal mammary artery may be grafted to the left anterior descending artery. (See *A less invasive alternative.*)

Before

When providing care to a patient about to undergo a CABG, assess the patient's cardiovascular status. Explain the procedure and its risks and benefits. Prepare him for postoperative care measures. (See *What the patient needs to know about a CABG,* page 96.)

After

After a CABG, perform the following care measures:

• Assess the patient's cardiovascular status.

Now I get it!

A less invasive alternative

Minimally invasive direct coronary artery bypass (MIDCAB) may offer benefits over a traditional coronary artery bypass graft (CABG). The MIDCAB is similar to a conventional CABG in that an internal mammary artery is used to bypass a blocked section of a coronary artery.

However, the MIDCAB doesn't require use of cardiopulmonary bypass, which reduces discomfort for the patient and decreases recovery time. In addition, the sternum isn't broken during the procedure, as it is with a CABG. The surgeon operates directly on the heart through a 4" to 4¾" (10- to 12-cm) long incision. The traditional CABG requires a 12" (30-cm) incision.

Advantages

The MIDCAB offers several advantages.
• It doesn't require a thoracotomy. A 3" (8-cm) incision is made for the permanent removal of a 2" (5-cm) section of rib for access.
• It doesn't require a bypass machine.
• Unlike in a CABG, the heart continues to beat during the procedure, except for approximately 10 minutes during graft surgery.
• It offers a quicker recovery time, compared with both CABG and percutaneous transluminal coronary angioplasty.
• It costs about a third less than a standard CABG.

Disadvantages

Despite its many advantages, the MIDCAB is associated with two key disadvantages.
• It's suitable only for patients who have one artery blocked so severely that angioplasty will fail.
• Cutting off the heart's blood supply for 10 minutes may raise the risk of a myocardial infarction.

Listen up!

What the patient needs to know about a CABG

Make sure the patient understands that a coronary artery bypass graft (CABG) won't cure CAD but that it will relieve the symptoms. The patient must still work to reduce controllable risk factors. Remind the patient to:
• lose weight. If overweight, the patient should limit caloric intake and exercise as much as possible and advisable.
• maintain a healthy diet. Remind the patient to limit his intake of salts, fats, and cholesterol.
• ease stress. If stress is a trigger for CAD symptoms, teach the patient stress reduction techniques, such as meditation and biofeedback.
• quit smoking.

• Monitor the patient's fluid status.
• Inspect the incisions.
• Be alert for arrhythmia, especially atrial fibrillation. Intervene as needed.
• Assess hemoglobin and arterial blood gas levels, hematocrit, partial thromboplastin time, and electrolyte levels.

Atrial fibrillation after a CABG

Atrial fibrillation usually occurs in paroxysms between the second and fifth postoperative days. The arrhythmia is probably directly related to the effects of surgery, such as pericarditis, changes in autonomic tone, cardioplegia, myocardial damage, and fluid shifts within the myocardium.

Management of atrial fibrillation after a CABG is initially directed at controlling the ventricular rate, but the ultimate goal is return to a sinus rhythm. The approach to therapy depends on several variables, including the duration of the arrhythmia. However, hemodynamic stability of the patient is the key issue.

Keep these points in mind when caring for a patient with atrial fibrillation after a CABG:

• Beta blockers or calcium channel blockers may prevent or terminate atrial fibrillation following a CABG.

• Class IA and III antiarrhythmics should be reserved for persistent or poorly tolerated episodes of atrial fibrillation.

• Elective cardioversion, either by direct current or with drugs, should be delayed as long as possible after surgery.

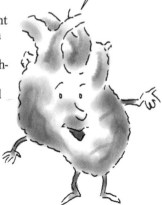

After I get a CABG, watch for arrhythmia, especially atrial fibrillation.

• Provide discharge teaching throughout the postoperative period.
• Encourage the patient to increase activity gradually.
• When the patient is discharged from the health care facility, remind him to monitor his risk factors for CAD.

Cardiac rehabilitation

By participating in a cardiac rehabilitation program, a patient with CAD can maintain fitness while minimizing the chance of experiencing another cardiac event. The patient typically starts rehabilitation as soon as his condition stabilizes.

Phases

Cardiac rehabilitation programs offer supervised exercise training, education, and support for the patient and family. Comprehensive programs involve three phases.

Phase I

The initial phase takes place in the hospital so that the patient can be closely monitored. During phase I, the patient participates in progressive self-care activities, ambulation, and exercise programs. The patient learns about CAD, risk factors, proper diet, drugs, and strategies for coping with psychosocial problems related to the condition.

Phase II

The second phase begins when the patient leaves the hospital and continues for about 8 weeks thereafter. Organized activities include educational programs, social events, and support groups. During phase II, give the patient three main goals:
• build strength gradually
• improve cardiovascular fitness
• gain confidence.

Phase III

Designed to improve the patient's general physical condition, phase III involves the patient's participation in an exercise program two or three times a week. The patient isn't monitored during these activities, but may exercise in a facility that offers emergency treatment and electrocardiogram testing. The patient monitors his own risk factors, such as high blood pressure or a high cholesterol level, and may attend educational classes.

Evaluating the program

When evaluating the outcome of your patient's participation in a cardiac rehabilitation program, consider the following:

• Does the patient understand the reason for treatment?

• Can the patient explain CAD risk factors, including the difference between those that can be controlled and those that can't?

• Does the patient understand ways to reduce risk factors and prevent or reduce the chance of future cardiac injury?

The three phases of cardiac rehabilitation progress steadily, helping the patient gain confidence along the way.

Quick quiz

1. PTCA opens coronary arteries by:
   A. removing plaque.
   B. compressing plaque.
   C. flushing plaque out of the vessel.

Answer: B. During a PTCA, a balloon-tipped catheter is placed into a stenosed coronary artery. Inflation of the balloon compresses the plaque, thereby widening the vessel lumen.

2. The purpose of implanting an intracoronary stent is to:
   A. prevent unstable angina.
   B. decrease the risk of restenosis.
   C. reduce myocardial oxygen demand.

Answer: B. Placement of an intracoronary stent may decrease the risk of restenosis.

3. Management of atrial fibrillation after a CABG is initially directed at:
   A. controlling the atrial rate.
   B. controlling the ventricular rate.
   C. maintaining renal perfusion.

Answer: B. Management of atrial fibrillation after a CABG is initially directed at controlling the ventricular rate, but the ultimate goal is a return to sinus rhythm.

4. Elective cardioversion for a patient having a CABG is usually done:
   A. during the operation.
   B. shortly after the operation.
   C. as long as possible after the operation.

Answer: C. Elective cardioversion, either by direct current or with drugs, should be delayed as long as possible after surgery.

Scoring

☆☆☆ If you answered all four questions correctly, congratulations! You've just graduated from the cardiac rehabilitation program with flying colors!

☆☆ If you answered three questions correctly, cool! You can now move up to the next phase of cardiac rehabilitation!

☆ If you answered fewer than three questions correctly, don't fret. Your cardiac rehabilitation program is designed to keep you healthy and movin' on up, no matter what!

5

CAD complications

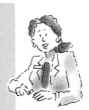

Key facts
- CAD can lead to emergency complications, such as MI and sudden cardiac arrest.
- Treatment for CAD, such as percutaneous transluminal coronary angioplasty, can also produce complications.
- Restenosis is the most common treatment-related complication of CAD.

Disease or treatment complications

Three main complications of coronary artery disease (CAD) or its treatment exist: myocardial infarction (MI), sudden cardiac arrest, and restenosis following percutaneous transluminal coronary angioplasty (PTCA).

Myocardial infarction

As CAD develops, blood flow to the myocardium decreases, either because of coronary artery spasm or because of increasing coronary artery occlusion with plaque. This decreased blood flow initially leads to angina pectoris, the classic symptom of CAD.

If angina isn't relieved or if CAD has deprived the heart of oxygen, ischemia (tissue injury) results. If the injury is left untreated, an MI may occur. In an MI, heart tissue dies due to lack of oxygen.

MI causes

Several factors can spark an MI. Atherosclerosis and severe coronary artery stenosis or spasm are the most common, but there are others, including coronary artery thrombosis or trauma that causes acute blood loss.

Less common factors involved in causing an MI include:
- coronary artery embolism
- dissecting aortic aneurysm
- neoplasm
- polyarteritis nodosa
- radiation therapy.

Sudden, severe pain

Unlike angina, MI pain lasts at least 20 minutes (and may last several hours) and is not relieved by rest. Look for:

> Lots of conditions can lead to an MI, though atherosclerosis and coronary artery stenosis are most common.

- chest pain that occurs suddenly
- pain that increases in severity
- pain in the lower substernal area
- pain that radiates to the neck, back, left arm, shoulder, or jaw.

Impending doom

During an MI, your patient may appear pale, diaphoretic, or light-headed, or be short of breath. Many patients also experience a sense of impending doom during an MI.

Watch out for the quiet ones

Not all MIs involve pain. Occasionally a patient shows other signs of MI — such as diaphoresis and pallor — but doesn't actually complain of pain. Only diagnostic tests such as an electrocardiogram (ECG) or cardiac enzyme levels indicate the occurrence of an MI.

Making sure

Although MI pain may initially resemble angina, definitive diagnosis requires a combination of assessments, including the patient's symptoms, cardiac enzyme levels, and 12-lead ECG changes.

Sudden cardiac arrest

Sudden cardiac arrest occurs mainly among men ages 45 to 69 and accounts for 500,000 deaths a year. In many cases, cardiac arrest is the first sign of heart disease.

VTach and then VFib

In many instances, sudden cardiac arrest is preceded by ventricular tachycardia and unconsciousness. The patient's condition then typically degenerates to ventricular fibrillation. The prognosis worsens the longer the patient is unconscious and the longer the heart is fibrillating.

Return of CAD risk factors

A patient at risk for sudden cardiac arrest typically has the same risk factors as a patient at risk for CAD. The patient may or may not have a history of MI. Other risk factors include:
- aortic stenosis
- atrioventricular block
- dilated or hypertrophic cardiomyopathy
- prolonged QT syndrome
- Wolff-Parkinson-White syndrome.

Restenosis

PTCA, a common treatment for CAD, can result in restenosis, a narrowing of recently opened blood vessels. Restenosis is one of the more common complications of PTCA. (See *Complications of percutaneous transluminal coronary angioplasty,* page 108.)

Although the number of other acute complications of PTCA have declined steadily in recent years, restenosis continues to occur at a steady rate. The cardinal symptom of restenosis is a return of angina within 6 months after PTCA.

Restenosis risk factors

Though in many cases restenosis occurs following PTCA, certain factors seem to increase the risk of this complication. These risk factors include:
• angioplasty performed on the proximal coronary artery segments or left anterior descending coronary artery
• diabetes mellitus
• large, complicated internal dissections

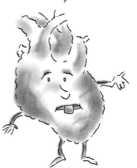

Just when you think my vessels are wide open — wham — restenosis sets in.

Complications of percutaneous transluminal coronary angioplasty

Complication	Signs and symptoms	Treatment
Coronary artery spasm This complication involves a spontaneous sustained contraction of the coronary artery, which causes ischemia and dysfunction of the heart muscle.	• Angina • Arrhythmias • Decreased blood pressure • Altered heart rate	Drugs, such as a calcium channel blocker or nitroglycerin
Dissection of coronary artery This complication occurs during the dilation of an artery and can lead to coronary artery rupture, cardiac tamponade, myocardial ischemia, MI, or death.	• Diaphoresis • Tachycardia • Hypotension	Immediate coronary artery bypass grafting
Hematoma This complication involves a localized collection of blood at the catheter insertion site.	• Bruising, swelling, and pain at insertion site	Pressure dressing and sandbag to prevent further bleeding; monitor site, vital signs, and peripheral pulses
Pseudoaneurysm This complication typically occurs as a result of blood vessel trauma, which disrupts the inner and medial layers of the vessel wall, allowing a channel to form within the wall.	• Similar to hematoma • Bruit over the puncture site	Ultrasound guided compression, if unsuccessfully repaired by a vascular surgeon

- progressive narrowing of coronary vessels before angioplasty
- recent onset of angina
- unstable angina before angioplasty
- use of an undersized or oversized angioplasty balloon.

Restenosis now...

Restenosis can be classified as acute or chronic, depending on how soon it occurs after the PTCA. Acute (or early) restenosis occurs shortly after PTCA and affects 2% to 6% of patients. Possible causes of acute restenosis include:

- occlusion from a large intimal flap
- sudden relaxation of the stretched, disease-free vessel wall opposite an eccentrically shaped plaque
- spasm of the coronary lumen wall
- thrombus associated with a large, curled intimal flap.

...or restenosis later

Chronic or late restenosis occurs within 6 months after angioplasty and affects 30% to 50% of the patients who undergo the procedure. Possible causes include:

> Hey, get the balloon size right, would ya? I don't want that restenosis thing again.

- balloon inflation pressure
- location of the angioplasty site
- multivessel involvement in the procedure
- use of anticoagulants or vasodilators.

Treating complications

In many cases, treating complications of CAD involves emergency, sometimes lifesaving, therapies directed at halting an MI, reversing sudden cardiac arrest, or relieving a restenosis.

Treating an MI

When a patient is suffering an MI, initial treatment focuses on reducing his pain and preventing further myocardial damage. Other treatments seek to maximize myocardial oxygenation, reduce myocardial oxygen demands, and help the patient maintain adequate cardiac output.

Immediate action

If a patient suffers an MI, immediate management should include obtaining a 12-lead ECG, placing the patient on bed rest, monitoring his heart rhythm, administering oxygen and I.V. fluids as ordered, and analyzing blood studies, especially cardiac enzyme and isoenzyme levels. Drug therapy also plays a key role in the treatment of a patient with an MI.

Drugs for an MI

Drug therapy for an MI focuses on reducing pain. Morphine and meperidine are examples of narcotic analgesics commonly used to treat an MI. Thrombolytics such as streptokinase are administered as soon as possible. These drugs can dissolve the clot in an artery occluded by a thrombus and thereby restore perfusion to the myocardium.

Other drugs adjust the heart's need for oxygen by increasing the supply of oxygen or reducing the heart's demand for it. Beta blockers, for instance, decrease myocardial oxygen demand. Nitroglycerin products increase myocardial oxygen supply and improve coronary artery perfusion.

Some MI drugs reduce the pain caused by an MI; others reduce my need for oxygen.

6-hour window for thrombolytics

Thrombolytic therapy can restore myocardial perfusion and prevent heart tissue from dying. This therapy is used when the patient's MI results from acute coronary thrombosis. The therapy is most effective when administered within 6 hours of the onset of an MI.

If not successfully treated, an MI can progress to additional, significant complications.

ABCs of PTCAs and CABGs

A PTCA or coronary artery bypass graft (CABG) can be used to restore blood flow through damaged coronary vessels. In a PTCA, the doctor inserts a balloon-tipped catheter into the artery to open a blockage or narrowing. During a CABG, a surgeon uses a healthy vessel to divert blood flow around a damaged or blocked artery.

Temporary measure

An intra-aortic balloon pump (IABP) displaces blood within the aorta, increasing the supply of oxygen-rich blood to the heart. An IABP can help temporarily relieve severe chest pain, stabilize the condition of a patient in cardiogenic shock, or stabilize the condition of a patient awaiting CABG surgery.

Treating sudden cardiac arrest

Treatment for sudden cardiac arrest depends on how long the patient has been unconscious and whether or not he has an underlying heart rhythm.

Stat!

For acute situations in which the patient has been unconscious for only a few minutes or less and the underlying rhythm is lethal, immediate defibrillation and administration of antiarrhythmics are generally required.

Semi-stat!

For repeated episodes of certain ventricular arrhythmias considered dangerous but not always lethal, an implantable cardioverter-defibrillator may be required for long-term control.

Treating restenosis

Restenosis is generally treated with a repeat balloon angioplasty in which the balloon is inflated for longer periods of time. Two other techniques are also gaining popularity:

> ### Battling illness
>
> ## Send in the stent
> The doctor may use various techniques to insert a stent, including:
> - inserting the stent under a fluoroscope
> - threading the stent to the angioplasty site
> - implanting the stent within the vessels.
>
> ### Not problem-free
> Although using a stent can help prevent restenosis, stent insertion involves other problems, such as the following:
> - The stent may block visibility during a percutaneous transluminal coronary angioplasty.
> - The doctor may miss the desired location when inserting a stent.
> - The device may slip out of position in the catheter delivery system.
> - The size of the stent and the way it appears on a radiographic monitor make it difficult to determine correct placement.

🖐 atherectomy, used to remove large intimal-medial flaps, a thrombus, or both

✌ intracoronary stenting, commonly used with initial angioplasty. (See *Send in the stent*.) Early studies suggest that stents decrease the risk of restenosis by about 50%.

Quick quiz

1. Factors that place the patient at risk for developing restenosis include:
   A. diabetes mellitus.
   B. smoking.
   C. history of rheumatic heart disease as a child.

Answer: A. The presence of diabetes mellitus puts the patient at an increased risk for restenosis.

2. The pain of an MI lasts a minimum of:
   A. 5 minutes.
   B. 20 minutes.
   C. 60 minutes.

Answer: B. Unlike angina, MI pain lasts for at least 20 minutes and isn't relieved by rest.

3. Complications of an MI include:
   A. atrial aneurysm.
   B. cardiogenic shock.
   C. endocarditis.

Answer: B. Cardiogenic shock is a complication of an MI; endocarditis and atrial aneurysm are not.

Scoring

☆☆☆ If you answered all three questions correctly, right on! You respond rapidly to complications and quick quizzes!

☆☆ If you answered two questions correctly, congratulations! There's nothing complicated about your quick quiz capabilities!

☆ If you answered fewer than two questions correctly, don't worry. These complications become less complicated after a review of this chapter.

6

Teaching patients with CAD

Key facts
♦ Teaching about CAD should emphasize lifestyle changes.
♦ Thoroughly explaining the diagnosis may help motivate the patient to take steps to prevent CAD's progress.
♦ Teaching should include a discussion of the wide range of available therapies and treatments.

Teaching about CAD

When teaching a patient about CAD, begin by discussing the four basic facts about the disease:

✌ Coronary arteries provide oxygenated blood to the heart.

✌ In patients who develop CAD, fatty plaques form along the inside walls of the coronary arteries.

These plaques can eventually decrease blood flow to the heart, robbing the heart of vital oxygen.

Without oxygen, the heart can suffer any of a variety of serious complications, including arrhythmia, heart failure, and myocardial infarction (MI).

Risk factors

Explain to your patient that a number of risk factors increase the chances that he'll develop CAD. People at high risk for CAD generally possess at least one risk factor, such as having reached age 55, and at least one less risky but contributing factor, such as being overweight.

To modify, or not to modify

These risk factors fall into two categories: nonmodifiable (unable to be changed) and modifiable (can potentially be changed).

Nonmodifiable risk factors include the patient's:
• age
• family history
• gender

- race.
  Modifiable risk factors include:
- high blood pressure
- diabetes mellitus
- obesity
- sedentary lifestyle
- elevated serum cholesterol levels
- smoking
- stress.

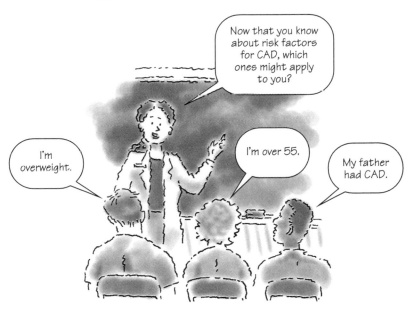

Signs and symptoms

Your patient needs to understand the importance of recognizing angina pectoris (chest pain with a cardiac origin) and the urgency in seeking medical treatment quickly.

Classic angina

Teach the patient that angina pectoris is the classic symptom of CAD. Angina results from inadequate blood flow to the heart. Inadequate blood flow prevents the heart from receiving enough oxygen, causing chest pain. Angina commonly occurs after physical exertion and is usually relieved by rest.

Diagnostic tests

Teach the patient that if he has a history of CAD-related symptoms such as angina and if he possesses significant CAD risk factors, he may undergo one or more diagnostic tests to determine if he has developed CAD. (See *Testing for CAD*.) Patients at high risk for CAD sometimes undergo tests to diagnose CAD even before they show any symptoms.

Listen up!

Testing for CAD

Explain to the patient that along with blood tests, he may undergo additional procedures to monitor the progress of CAD. Those tests include:
- 12-lead electrocardiogram (ECG)
- exercise stress test
- coronary angiography.

Catching the rhythm

For the 12-lead ECG, instruct the patient to lie still while a technician applies wires and gel patches to his chest. Tell him that this quick, painless test will show disturbances in heart rhythm as well as areas of damaging myocardial oxygen deprivation.

It's just like riding a bike

For the exercise stress test, explain to the patient that he'll exercise (either on a bicycle or treadmill) while the hospital staff records the electrical activity of his heart. Tell him that the test reveals evidence of insufficient blood flow to the heart.

You're positively glowing

For the coronary angiography, explain to the patient that a doctor will thread a catheter into the patient's heart and evaluate pressure readings and oxygen saturation. Then, the patient will be injected with a contrast medium to show heart chambers and structures under a fluoroscope. Explain that this test reveals much about the coronary arteries and helps to determine the presence or the extent of CAD.

Tests, tests, and more tests

Tests used to diagnose CAD include:
- 12-lead electrocardiogram (ECG)
- cardiac enzyme levels, which detect the presence of heart damage
- coronary angiography, to determine vessel patency
- exercise stress test
- serum lipid profile.

Teaching about lifestyle changes

Explain to the patient that lifestyle changes are critical for preventing CAD and managing the disease once it has developed. The patient may need to make changes in diet, exercise habits, smoking habits, and stress management.

Exercise

Teach the patient that regular exercise can prevent CAD from developing or at least impede its progression. Stress the importance of daily exercise, and help him find ways to incorporate exercise into his normal routine. Look for activities that the patient enjoys and can perform fairly easily such as walking.

Walking and talking

Teach the patient to apply the "talk test" while exercising. The patient should exercise to the point of slight breathlessness but still be able to talk easily. Encourage the patient to exercise at this level for 30 minutes every day or as close to every day as possible.

Chest pain = stop

Remind the patient to exercise cautiously. The patient should increase activity slowly under the supervision of his primary care provider. He should also balance activity with rest to prevent excess fatigue. Emphasize that if chest pain develops, he should cease activity immediately. (See *Making whoopee,* page 124.)

Stress

Teach the patient stress reduction techniques, such as deep breathing, progressive relaxation, and meditation. Explain that although many events are out of the patient's control, how the patient reacts to

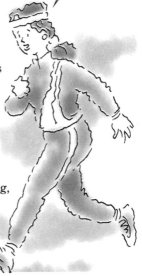

OK, the patient can walk the walk and talk the talk. But can he do both at once?

Making whoopee

A patient with CAD may have concerns regarding sexual activity. Listen to his concerns, and teach him how and when he can safely resume sexual activity.

Take this pill...

Tell the patient to take antianginal drugs before sex and to avoid sex for at least 2 hours after meals.

...but not this one

Warn the patient that he shouldn't take sildenafil (Viagra) if he's taking a nitrate. Nitrate therapy is an absolute contraindication during sildenafil therapy. Concurrent use of sildenafil and a nitrate can cause life-threatening hypotension.

those events plays a major role in reducing stress and workload on the heart. In addition, encourage the patient to develop relationships with friends and family members who can provide support in times of stress. Other patients with CAD can offer a valuable source of support during high stress periods.

More on coping...

Other ways to cope with stress include exercising, limiting caffeine and alcohol intake, cutting back on or quitting smoking, and learning to accept things that can't be changed.

Diet

Diet modifications can reduce the risk of developing CAD, prevent its progression, and improve overall health. Patient teaching about diet should focus on reducing saturated fats and increasing fiber intake.

Forego those four-egg omelets

Teach the patient to decrease the amount of saturated fat in his diet by:
• avoiding red meat or using only lean cuts of red meat, such as round or sirloin

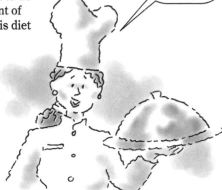

Allow me to recommend a delicious low-fat diet, starring a lovely lean breast of chicken, broiled to perfection without saturated fats.

- avoiding processed meats, such as cold cuts or hot dogs
- avoiding whole milk products, and switching to nonfat milk products
- avoiding saturated tropical oils and substituting olive oil or canola oil
- removing the skin from poultry before cooking
- broiling, baking, or poaching chicken, turkey, fish, or lean cuts of meat, rather than frying
- eating no more than three egg yolks a week, including yolks in prepared foods
- eating fresh, frozen, or canned fruit
- eating grains and breads such as plain rice, pasta, English muffins, bagels, or tortillas.

Pass the fiber, please

Explain to the patient that he should increase his fiber intake to help reduce the risk of constipation, a common adverse reaction of several antianginal drugs.

Smoking

If the patient smokes, discuss the need to quit smoking. Encourage him to seek a support group in the area to help him give up smoking.

Transdermal nicotine eases the transition

Explain that several transdermal nicotine systems are now available. These systems allow the individual to gradually decrease the amount of nicotine received each day, lessening the severity of adverse reactions related to smoking and improving compliance.

Teaching about drugs

Comprehensive teaching about cardiac drugs encourages the patient to comply with therapy and may help to prevent adverse reactions.

Heart Drugs 101

With any drug the patient is prescribed, make sure he understands:
• when to take the drug (time)
• how much to take (amount)
• how often to take it (frequency)
• for how long (duration).
Explain the drug's adverse effects, and remind the patient that he should never abruptly stop taking a heart drug without first notifying his primary care provider.

Listen up!

Stand up slowly

While taking vasodilators, the patient may experience orthostatic hypotension. To avoid this adverse reaction, teach him to:
• rise slowly from a lying to a sitting position
• place both feet firmly on the floor before standing
• lie or sit immediately if he feels light-headed or dizzy
• avoid sudden or abrupt shifts while walking
• report episodes of dizziness.

Heart Drugs 102

In addition, teach the patient to:
• report adverse drug reactions to the doctor (see *Stand up slowly*)
• call the doctor before taking over-the-counter drugs
• establish a daily drug routine that fits his lifestyle
• measure the heart rate and blood pressure once or twice a week. Have him record the results in a journal.

In addition, make sure the patient knows what interactions are possible with other drugs.

Teaching about procedures

The most common procedure used to treat CAD is percutaneous transluminal coronary angioplasty (PTCA), also known as balloon angioplasty. PTCA offers an alternative to bypass surgery and can improve blood flow through the coronary artery by enlarging the diseased artery's lumen.

Pre-PTCA

Thoroughly explain PTCA and its risks to the patient. Tell him:

• he'll be awake during the procedure and that he'll need to take deep breaths and cough when asked

• he may feel flushed when the contrast medium is first injected but this feeling will pass

• he must report allergies to shellfish, iodine, or contrast dyes

• he'll have an I.V. line and take nothing by mouth for at least 6 hours before the procedure

• his vital signs and heart rhythm will be monitored during the procedure.

No place like home

Home care after a PTCA

When the patient is ready to leave the hospital after a percutaneous transluminal coronary angioplasty (PTCA), discuss home care measures with him. Explain his drug regimen, and advise him to:

• apply pressure over the I.V. site in the groin when coughing or sneezing and avoid bearing down during bowel movements

• apply pressure to the arterial puncture site site and call his primary care provider if bleeding or bruising is noted at the site

• notify his primary care provider regarding chest pain not relieved by his prescribed drug

• avoid lifting more than 10 lb (4.5 kg) for 2 to 3 weeks, until the puncture and angioplasty sites have healed

• keep all follow-up appointments

• follow required lifestyle changes.

Post-PTCA

Tell the patient he'll need to continue therapy with heparin, nitroglycerin, or other drug, as ordered. (See *Home care after a PTCA.*) He should also expect to:

• maintain bed rest, with the head of the bed elevated no more than 15 degrees

• undergo frequent monitoring of vital signs, fluid intake, and peripheral pulses
• undergo frequent assessment of the puncture site, which will be covered by a dressing and sandbag
• continue receiving I.V. fluids.

Teaching about surgery

The main surgical treatment for CAD is a coronary artery bypass graft (CABG). Explain to the patient that a CABG can restore blood flow to a damaged heart by bypassing a blockage in the coronary artery.

Tell the patient that the surgeon removes a portion of a healthy vessel from another part of the body and grafts it in place, from above the blocked portion to below. Blood then circulates through the graft rather than the blocked artery.

Pre-CABG

Explain the equipment used in a CABG, and arrange a tour of the intensive care unit, if possible, to help increase the patient's comfort level. In addition, discuss:
• consent forms

No place like home

Home care after a CABG

When the patient is ready to leave the hospital, explore home care measures with him. Explain his drug regimen, and discuss:
• wound care
• coughing and deep-breathing exercises
• proper responses to chest pain
• warning signs that necessitate medical attention
• importance of maintaining follow-up visits.

Everyday activities
Remember to also discuss:
• ways to manage bathing and showering activities
• importance of daily weight measurements
• exercise and activity tolerance
• activity limitations (for example, with regard to lifting and driving)
• travel and work restrictions
• other lifestyle changes and cardiac risks.

• importance of maintaining nothing-by-mouth status
• preoperative medications and procedures
• spiritual needs or other sources of support the patient desires. (See *Home care after a CABG*.)

Getting connected

CAD sites on the Internet

For more information on CAD, check these Web sites.

American Heart Association
www.amhrt.org
Written primarily for patients, this library of information links to sites about the heart and provides basic information in easy-to-understand language.

Cardiovascular Research Institute of Southern California
www.cvri.com
The Cardiovascular Research Institute of Southern California is a tertiary clinical research facility. This site provides a review of research findings as well as the clinical trials of various treatments for CAD.

Empower Health Corporation
www.drkoop.com
This site, from former U.S. Surgeon General Dr. C. Everett Koop, offers information on CAD-related topics, such as wellness and prevention, physical findings and symptoms, and making a diagnosis. Check this site for patient-teaching information about CAD prevention.

Heart and Stroke Association of Canada
www.hsf.ca
Oriented towards patients, this site provides a basic overview of cardiovascular disease, a series of fact sheets on specific topics, health news and statistics, and a review of the latest research. Also contains a section on how diet can reduce the risk of heart disease.

(continued)

CAD sites on the Internet *(continued)*

Heart Information Network

www.heartinfo.com

Visitors to this site can obtain heart information news, frequently asked questions, and links to other sites. They can also determine their risk for developing heart disease. For patients with stories to share, there's a section for posting personal experiences.

Mayo Health Clinic

www.mayohealth.org

An informative resource covering many aspects of heart disease, the Mayo Health Clinic site features a range of reference articles, quizzes, Ask the Doctor, and links to related sites.

National Heart, Lung, and Blood Association

www.nhlbi.nih.gov/nhlbi/cardio

A general fact sheet for patients concerning heart disease, this site also provides a list of sources for additional information.

New York Online Access to Health

www.noah.cuny.edu

Sponsored cooperatively by the City University of New York, The New York Academy of Medicine, and other organizations, New York Online Access to Health (NOAH) contains little original content but is a good directory of other Internet resources for information about heart disease. Most of the information is available in Spanish.

Post-CABG

Tell the patient to expect frequent assessment and monitoring of his vital signs, fluid intake, ventilation, incision, and drainage tubes. Explain that he'll need to cough and breathe deeply regularly to prevent pneumonia and atelectasis, and that he'll need to gradually increase his activity level, according to his primary care provider's plan.

Quick quiz

1. A patient with CAD who feels chest pain while exercising should:

    A. stop exercising immediately.

    B. slow down his pace until the pain stops.

    C. continue unless the pain be comes debilitating.

Answer: A. A patient who feels chest pain while exercising should stop immediately and notify his doctor.

2. When teaching the patient about PTCA, ask if he is allergic to:

    A.   codeine.

    B.   molds.

    C.   shellfish.

Answer: C. Shellfish contain iodine and could herald an allergy to the dye used during the procedure.

3. Explain to your patient having a CABG that, after surgery, he'll need to cough and breathe deeply to prevent:

    A.   arrhythmia and hypotension.

    B.   pneumonia and atelectasis.

    C.   stroke and renal failure.

Answer: B. Explain that he'll need to cough and deep-breathe regularly to prevent pneumonia and atelectasis.

Scoring

☆☆☆   If you answered all three questions correctly, congratulations! You're our CAD Teacher of the Year!

☆☆   If you answered two questions correctly, all right! Step up to the nearest chalkboard and teach away!

☆   If you answered fewer than two questions correctly, no biggie. We think you have what it takes to teach terrifically!

Index

A

Acute coronary insufficiency, 47-49. *See also* Angina.
Aerobic exercise, 40
African Americans
    coronary artery disease in, 23
Age, as risk factor, 23
Anaerobic exercise, 40-41
Aneurysm, dissecting, as risk factor, 3
Angina, 47-58
    blood flow and, 49
    causes of, 53
    crescendo, 47-49
    differential diagnosis of, 54
    history of, 47-58
    identification of, 50-52, 55
    intractable, 52
    location of, 48i
    nocturnal, 52
    pain of, 49
    preinfarction, 47-49
    Prinzmetal's, 49, 52-53
    questions about, 55
    refractory, 52
    stable, 47, 50-51
    in stress test, 63
    teaching about, 120
    types of, 47-53

Angina *(continued)*
    unstable, 47, 50-51
    variant, 49, 52-53
Angiography, coronary, 66-69, 122
Angioplasty, restenosis after, 16
Antilipemics, 76-79
Aorta, 10
Apolipoproteins, 29
Assessment, 45-69
    diagnostic procedures in, 62-69. *See also* Diagnostic procedures.
    diagnostic tests in, 60-62
    health history in, 45-58. *See also* Health history.
    physical examination in, 58-60
Atherectomy, 114
Atherosclerosis, 2
    development of, 12-15
    stages of, 12-15
Atherosclerotic plaque, 11i
    cracking of, 87
    eccentric, 16
    formation of, 12i-15i
    rupture of, 8
Atrial fibrillation, after coronary artery bypass graft, 96-98

B

Bed rest, 74-75
Bepridil hydrochloride (Vascor), 81

i refers to an illustration; t refers to a table.

i refers to an illustration; t refers to a table.

i refers to an illustration; t refers to a table.

i refers to an illustration; t refers to a table.

i refers to an illustration; t refers to a table.

i refers to an illustration; t refers to a table.

i refers to an illustration; t refers to a table.